ALL IN THE MIND

Victoria Martin

chipmunkapublishing
the mental health publisher

Victoria Martin

All rights reserved, no part of this publication may be reproduced by any means, electronic, mechanical photocopying, documentary, film or in any other format without prior written permission of the publisher.

> Published by
> Chipmunkapublishing
> PO Box 6872
> Brentwood
> Essex CM13 1ZT
> United Kingdom

http://www.chipmunkapublishing.com

Copyright © Victoria Martin 2009

Edited by Charlotte Tipping

Chipmunkapublishing gratefully acknowledge the support of Arts Council England.

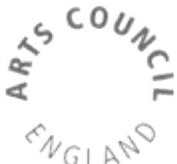

ALL IN THE MIND

INTRODUCTION

It is not politically correct to use terms like 'barking mad,' when describing someone with a mental illness, but it does sum up the reaction you can expect if you are brave enough to admit that you are a sufferer! With that in mind I am writing this account under a pseudonym - and hope that you will find some strength from the knowledge that we all have idiosyncrasies and that it is only the degree to which they affect our lives that separates the 'normal' from the 'mentally ill'.

From the perspective of a 'normal' person it is easy to argue the illogical actions of a person who is mentally ill – but from the perspective of someone who is mentally ill it is frustrating and embarrassing to have your inability to carry out perfectly ordinary tasks questioned.

For years I had witnessed family members suffering with 'bad nerves' and I became somewhat blasé about it. Although I sympathised and empathised with them I was mainly an 'outsider' looking in with only a basic understanding of what they could and could not do. Very little thought actually went into how they really felt - until I, too, began to suffer.

It is with my 'normal' views still etched in my memory that I have decided to give an account from both points of view in an effort to shorten the gap between what is regarded as 'normal' and 'not normal' in relation to mental health.

All names have been changed to protect the identities of all the people portrayed within these pages.

ALL IN THE MIND

CHAPTER 1

My father had, what was commonly referred to as, a 'nervous breakdown' when he was in his fifties. This was my first experience of mental illness and it was confusing.

I must have been very young, because he was 48 when I was born, and my main memory consists of him in the kitchen, washing the dishes, whilst my sister and I argued. I remember his shoulders going up and down and for a moment we thought that he was laughing and began laughing ourselves – only to see him turning to face us in tears.

For a man who always seemed to be in good spirits – and possessed a somewhat dry sense of humour – this shocked and surprised us. I do not remember ever having seen him cry before and felt confused if not a little alarmed.

An older sibling tried to explain that our father was not very well and advised us to give him some space – but we were even more confused by this because he did not look ill. They probably tried to explain further – that he was ill 'inside' and it did not show up in the same way as a broken leg – but I really cannot remember because I was too far removed from it to really understand.

That is the problem with mental illness. It often does not produce the same feelings of understanding and compassion as a broken leg or a visible injury.

They are identifiable problems that do not have a stigma attached to them. It is acceptable to admit that you cannot go somewhere because you have a broken leg – but who wants to admit that it is their nerves that makes it difficult for them to get around? Unless you have suffered problems yourself it is very difficult to understand something that is 'all in the mind'.

When my sister, Penny, accompanied him, to have his prescription made up in the local pharmacy, she was mortified when he wanted reassurance that his new medication would be as effective as the old one. She remembers thinking that they could have been giving him a packet of sweets - just as long as they assured him that they would do the job!

So there you have three typical examples of how people react – confused, shocked and embarrassed. But the main problem, really, is a lack of understanding. We were ignorant and as such we unable to comprehend how he felt.

There is a lot of ignorance surrounding the subject of mental health. People are regarded as either 'normal' or 'mentally ill' – but the truth is that you can have mental health problems and be totally sane. To suffer from a mental illness does not make you necessarily 'mad'- and, if you are currently lucky enough not to have a mental health

ALL IN THE MIND

issue do not assume that you, or someone you know, will never be affected by one.

Fast forward a few years and Penny was showing signs of mental illness herself – although it would be several more years before she would acknowledge the fact. Her problems started with missing school. At first it was an 'identifiable' illness – chicken pox or some childhood complaint - but it soon developed into a real fear that surfaced when she had to return to school.

This was not just a case of feeling nervous – this was intense anxiety that would result in an upset stomach and vomiting. But no one seemed to recognise the fact – at that stage I guess I probably did not recognise it either – which meant that the Truant Officer (School Bobby) was a frequent visitor.

As an 'outsider' at this point I can admit that at first I just thought that it was an excuse because she did not like school. I cannot say, in all honesty, that I understood how she felt or really believed that she was 'ill'. I would find her outside with her friends and point out that if she had not been well enough to go to school then she should not be out 'playing' now. She would invariably promise that she would go to school the next day – and sometimes she would try.

Because she was quiet in school she was picked on for being 'snooty' – and there is no doubt that the verbal bullying, that she experienced, did nothing to alleviate her problems – but it was not the bullying that really initiated the problem. Spending so much time away from school alienated her from her peers and it is this, I suspect, that caused the chasm to develop. But this created a vicious circle – she did not want to go to school but she would get pressured into going and then her classmates would make nasty comments so that she would not want to go to school again.

The school referred her to the school psychologist for counselling but this did not help because she did not want to go to the school in order to talk to him. She also thought that it was pointless because she could not explain why she felt the way that she did. How could she make people understand when she did not understand it herself? The doctor prescribed medication – but, having witnessed the effect of our father's dependency on pills, she was reluctant to take them. I remember being prescribed them myself so maybe I was not as 'normal', back then, as I would like to believe.

Our parents tried to persuade her to go to school - and even resorted to bribery by buying her a kitten in an effort to coax her - but to no avail. When she attempted to take an overdose, in an effort to avoid or to possibly, highlight the problem - the doctors had to acknowledge that forcing her to go to school was not the answer.

When I think back to that time I recall conversations where I would try to get her to talk to

ALL IN THE MIND

me – to explain why the thought of going to school made her feel so ill. I remember that she would say that she could not bear the thought of going through the school gates. Tellingly it was the 'thought' that made her feel ill – more often than not when we walked to school together she would feel ill all the way there (and worse as we approached the school gates) – but once inside she generally felt 'ok'. Ok is probably an overstatement – but she could cope.

As she got older, however, the cause of the problem had been whittled down to 'people'. She hates to drive but is fond of saying that she would be fine if there were no other cars on the road. What she really means, she explained, is that she would be fine if there were no other *people* on the road.
That may sound a little like agoraphobia – but, for reasons I will come to later, I do not think that that is the case.

Driving lessons were a traumatic experience for her. Her stomach would be upset and she would feel sick – and then there was the increased heartbeat and the sweaty palms to deal with. This was fear. She was no worse on her driving test really – and seven years after passing her driving test she is still no better.

This 'people' phobia basically makes personal contact very difficult for her. She hates meeting new people and will avoid it if at all possible. Unfortunately it even affects her ability to use the telephone. When the persistent ringing of her telephone began to irritate me I offered to answer it – but she argued that whoever it was might want to speak to her and, as she couldn't speak to anyone on the telephone, it would be pointless for me to answer it.

Irrationally, once the telephone stopped ringing she would be plagued with concerns over who it could have been and whether or not it was important. As you can guess this was in the days before that wonderful invention '1471'. I would be sympathetic, to a certain degree, but mainly I would be of no real help by pointing out that she could alleviate these worries by simply picking up the receiver. She would rightly point out that if she were able to do so she would have done! But I did not understand. The persistent ringing would make me feel anxious and I could not imagine that leaving it ringing could make her feel better.

This inability to answer the telephone resulted in the invention of a 'code' ring that would enable her to know who was on the other end. Only her immediate family (husband and son) knew this ring so she could answer it with relative ease. But it did not help her if anyone else tried to telephone. When '1471' came into being it allowed her to write down the caller's number so that her husband could return the call when he returned home. It was not ideal - but it was an improvement on wondering who the caller had been!

ALL IN THE MIND

Feeling nervous or anxious is a natural emotion and one that we all feel from time to time. It is only when you feel anxious or nervous for no reason – or these feelings are heightened beyond the 'norm' – that they become a problem. I began to feel anxious, outside of the normal scope of things, but still managed to maintain that I was 'ok'. If my sister was feeling inadequate and unable to cope I would feel even more 'ok' about my 'little quirks' – at least I was not *that* bad!

I remember us discussing her anxiety levels and me, in my ignorance, nodding and agreeing that I too sometimes felt like that but I 'didn't give in to it'. I must have reiterated this point a few times because finally she said: "It's not a matter of giving in to it. When you feel that bad you have no choice."

The irony is that there was no one who knew, better than she did how illogical her actions were. It did not take a genius to realise that nothing bad would happen if she answered the telephone – and surely answering the telephone had to be better than worrying about who was calling – but being logical had nothing to do with her inability to pick up that receiver.

Monica has suffered severe panic attacks that have had a paralysing effect on her. I recall an occasion that we were going on a night out when suddenly, and without any warning, she began to hyperventilate to such an extent, that she had to sit on the pavement until she recovered. Afterwards she was embarrassed and tried to make a joke out of it but it was evident that this was a real problem. Talking about it eventually helped her to come to terms with it but the most debilitating thing about it was that she never knew when it was going to happen.

My sister admitted that she too had suffered panic attacks. She would wake up at night with her heart and pulse racing and with the certainty that she was about to die.

It was whilst listening to their discussion that I realised how frustrated and embarrassed they felt. But, I realised, that although they shared similar feelings each could deal with different things. One preferred to be on her own – she could walk for miles on her own but felt more likely to 'panic' if she was in company. The other preferred to be in company – the prospect of going anywhere on her own was terrifying for her.

We were back at the realisation that no one knew better than they did how illogical their actions were. If I found it bizarre, that my sister could refuse to answer a ringing phone - and then spend the next half an hour worrying over who the caller had been - it was nothing to how frustrated and annoyed she was with herself. If I found it a little confusing to have Monica dropping to the floor, because she was physically unable to move another step, then, again it was nothing to the embarrassment and frustration that she felt.

ALL IN THE MIND

I think somewhere in the back of my mind I thought that I was lucky. Two of my acquaintances had 'problems' and I was 'ok'. I would try to understand and be supportive but their worries and anxieties were alien to me. I do not think that I ever really imagined that I could develop problems myself.

CHAPTER 2

So far I have mentioned three different people and given an indication of their problems and how I perceived them. I feel that it is important to give a varied account of all the people that I know and the problems that they have encountered, to raise awareness that it is far from 'rare'.

Now I would like to introduce Trudy. To all intents and purposes she has a confident and outgoing personality and is one of the least likely people you would expect to admit to having problems with their mental health. It was whilst we were there, having a Christmas drink one year, that my perceptions were about to change in more ways than one.

The conversation came around to panic attacks and people's general inability to cope with certain situations. I had nothing to contribute as I felt I was 'ok' – then Trudy admitted to having a few 'peculiarities' of her own. She declined invitations to go to her neighbours' houses because she did not feel that she could relax – she explained that if she invited people to her home she could 'disappear' upstairs, briefly, if it got too much for her. She then admitted that she took to lying on the landing for a few minutes when things got too bad.

I think that the main problem, at this time, was that I could perfectly understand her not wanting to accept invitations from her neighbours and declining offers seemed a reasonable course of

ALL IN THE MIND

action. I may not have fully understood why she resorted to lying down on the landing but I did not see it as a major problem!

When I pointed this out it became evident that although I saw nothing wrong with this my companions did. They could empathise with Trudy but did not feel that they needed to 'pretend' that her feelings were normal – any more than they pretended that their own behaviour could be regarded normal.

I became quite worried about this and as the discussion continued I had to accept that I had a few 'peculiarities' of my own. Maybe my willingness to accept other people's 'quirks', as normal, was a way of validating my own behaviour?

My sister pointed out that I had had a few problems helping her hang out some laundry – what she meant was that she had multi-coloured pegs and I 'needed' to use two pegs of the same colour for each item of clothing. I did not view this as a problem – in fact I thought I was being organised as it looked so much neater than using a combination of colours – but the way the others viewed this piece of news was much more telling.

In truth I had half acknowledged that I had a few problems of my own – but it was a bit of a blow to discover that other people were becoming aware of it! I am not entirely sure when I first realised it but I found myself adjusting the washing on the line so that the clothes were in size order. My husband's first, then mine, then my sons' – eldest first then the youngest.

If I took out an item of clothing that should have already been hung further up the line, I would move all the washing down to provide a space for it. If I picked up something belonging to my youngest son, it would go back in the basket until I was ready to peg it out.

But that was not all. As I have already mentioned I had to have two pegs, of the same colour, on each item of clothing so hanging out the laundry could take almost twice as long as it should have done whilst I searched for matching pegs. But I had also developed a problem with people.

I did not actually acknowledge it as such, for a long time, but I found myself peeping out into the garden to check if my neighbours were outside first. From this admission you might assume that I disliked my neighbours or had problems with them – but that is not the case. I have always gotten along well with them. The simple truth is that I just cannot face people sometimes. It has nothing to do with the person and everything to do with how I feel on any given day.

Why? I honestly do not know. Logically I cannot think of a reason. What do I think will happen? They will say 'Hello!' and a conversation will ensue – big deal! But on days when I cannot handle talking to people this seems like a very big deal. I have dried clothes inside, on a perfectly nice day,

ALL IN THE MIND

to avoid going outside. If anyone else admitted to this I would find it bizarre – I would understand it but I would recognise it as bizarre behaviour and I would ask them why and try to be logical about it – but logic does not help.

Actually that brings me to a very interesting point. Phobias are illogical. We all know this and take some comfort from the fact that we do not have any strange phobias like cotton reels or wool – but think for a moment about what you are afraid of. If it is cotton reels or wool I apologise for calling it a strange phobia and you have my deepest sympathy.

Imagine what you are really afraid of. Ok, if it is a 'real' fear, like heights for example, you could have a valid reason for being afraid. But, the chances are it is a typical one likes snakes or spiders. Now most of the snakes and spiders in this country are not poisonous so being afraid of them is illogical – but it does not make the fear any less real, does it?

In fact the chances are that whatever you are afraid of, there is no logical reasoning behind it. If you were to try to explain what makes you feel so loathe to face it, you will probably feel as frustrated and embarrassed as the person you are trying to convince. That should give you an idea of how it feels to know that you should be able to answer a ringing phone, for example, whilst at the same time be unable to 'face' it.

I found a way around my problem with pegs though – I bought wooden ones! But I still cannot persuade myself to hang out the washing in any other order. Actually, as my oldest son is now the second biggest in the family, his clothes go next to his father's. I still maintain that it looks tidier! It does not take me as long to hang out the washing now, either. I sort it out, into size order, before I go out into the garden! And if that means I have a problem I'm prepared to put up with it!

Whilst my sister battled with her inability to answer the telephone I had to fight with my urge to pick it up. I reasoned that it was an irritation that I could well do without – but in reality it was just another side of the same coin. A ringing telephone is a nuisance – but I am now in the position where my sister has spent most of her adult life, unable to answer the call.

That is not strictly true – I answer the telephone at work and have to make calls too – it is only at home that I choose to ignore it. This may sound strange - especially after my previous reaction to my sister's refusal to answer it - but I will try to explain.

At work I will generally delay picking up the phone knowing that the irritating sound will soon result in someone else answering it! Then, if the call is for me, the person's name and their reason for calling, is generally relayed by my colleague. I am then forearmed so to speak. If everyone else is busy, my conscience – not to mention my reluctance, to draw

ALL IN THE MIND

attention to my aversion to the phone – gets the better of me and I answer it myself.

At home we have had a lot of 'cold calls' from companies trying to interest us in a loan. My husband is out a lot so these calls result in them trying to pressure me (despite my statements that my husband deals with all that), or they hang up after declining to leave a message. I do not regard my choice to ignore these calls as a problem. I dial that wonderful little invention '1471' and decide whether or not to return the call – nine times out of ten the number is withheld and I have avoided another nuisance call.

If I leave that statement as it stands you will be forgiven for assuming that I really do not have a problem. I am quite adept at omitting things and giving misleading information – which my sister is becoming quite adept at recognising!

The truth is that my choice to ignore the ringing telephone is only half of the story. This does not explain my reluctance to *make* calls or why I make myself ill when I need to answer the telephone. I make calls in work – but again I will try to avoid it. If it is not urgent I will write instead – but if I really have to make a call I 'psyche' myself up for a while before hand.

At home I do not use the phone at all unless necessary. I will put off until tomorrow what I cannot face today – if I have to make calls I 'psyche' myself up and then dial the number quickly before thinking too much about it. It is not a pleasant feeling hearing the evidence that it is ringing on the other end and the temptation to hang up, before they answer, is almost overwhelming.

I would actually prefer to answer a ringing telephone than to make a call – which makes no sense. When the phone rings half of the problem is I do not know who is on the other end of the line. But when I make a call I do know (roughly) who is going to answer so this should be easier – but it is not.

What if I have to answer a call? I can. I am not comfortable about it but I can – depending on my state of mind. My sister uses the same ringing 'code' to call me as she still uses herself. Knowing her ring is a relief and I have no problem answering it. We are really close but at the moment I cannot bring myself to telephone her – and I know that sounds ridiculous. Hearing that sound, on the phone, is enough to raise my anxiety levels to an uncomfortable degree.

Anxiety is a terrible thing. Think of a time when you felt sick to your stomach. When you felt 'frightened' and just could not shake it. Did you have a reason to be afraid and anxious? I kind of hope you did – because fear and anxiety are natural emotions and it is normal to experience them when the situation dictates. But what if you had no reason to feel that way?

ALL IN THE MIND

I have had a few anxiety attacks and, at first, they were typically regarding my sons. I am a worrier and once the clock face shows the time that they should be indoors, I begin to get that feeling of dread in the pit of my stomach. I pace up and down and am very conscious of my breathing and find myself trying to swallow my fear. At this point I am absolutely convinced that my son (whichever one is late) is lying in a ditch somewhere and the police will be arriving at my door to break the news, any second now.

As soon as they walk through the door – with the excuse that their watch stopped or the chain came off their bike – I am relieved and mentally shake myself not to allow myself to get into such a state again. But it feels very real – like a premonition almost – and to ignore it would be like trying to quell the urge to comfort a crying child. I may be wrong but I would say that this is a normal reaction to anxiety.

As I say, I had a few anxiety attacks relating to my sons, but approximately two years ago I began to experience these episodes for no apparent reason. You may think I had no reason to feel so anxious about my sons arriving home late but that is beside the point.

I was feeling low and decided to make an appointment to see the doctor. On the morning of the appointment I felt a little nervous but nothing more. Half way to the surgery I had that awful feeling of dread and grew very conscious of my breathing. I felt afraid but did not know why – I was literally in tears and could not walk another step. It must have lasted a minute or so at most but it seemed much longer – it took some time to regulate my breathing.

Due to a thyroid problem the doctor told me that I am prone to depression and suggested another blood test. A telephone call, a few days later, confirmed a 'normal' result and that was the end of it. But it has happened several times since – and, just when I had resigned myself to having an anxiety attack, each time I am on my way to the surgery, I recently visited with no ill effects!

It is a cruel illness. You never know when it will strike and how it will affect you. Just when you think you have gotten it beat it will strike you down without warning – leaving you feeling worse than before because you convince yourself that you are 'ok'.

ALL IN THE MIND

CHAPTER 3

Thinking about the decline in my mental health is both embarrassing and frightening. I had regarded myself as 'normal' for so long that it was quite a profound moment when I admitted to myself that I had a problem.

Of course admitting it to myself was a breakthrough moment – but I do not think that I would have reached that moment, at the time that I did, if my sister had not prompted me. She made it easy to admit, at least on a basic level, that I had mental health issues of my own.

But that was really not as much help as it at first appeared. It is easy to assume that once you have made that big leap – by admitting you have a problem – it is plane sailing from there on in. But you would be wrong.

The trouble is it is not a typical illness. Everyone who has had chicken pox will agree that the itching drove them crazy. They will probably be able to point out the odd scar, or two, as a reminder that they were not always able to control the urge to scratch that itch. But with mental health issues you are hardly likely to find two people who feel the same.

On paper it can look like two people have exactly the same symptoms – but the physical manifestations will not always be the same and the sufferers are very unlikely to be able to do the same things.

My sister and I share the same aversion to the telephone. But I work in an environment that forces me to come into contact with it on a regular basis. My sister's anxiety levels noticeably rise if she just thinks about my job. She could not do it – despite sharing much of the same qualifications – and she can probably not imagine how I cope.

Thinking back, it surprised me to note that I probably had an aversion to the telephone several years earlier. My sister lived near our mother, at that time, and although I generally telephoned her prior to visiting – to check that she was not going out – I began to just 'chance it'. I reasoned that if she was not in I could always visit my mother instead.

When she moved I could no longer use this excuse. At first I would telephone to check that she was in – but then I would decide to 'risk it'. Typically I did not view this as a problem, and reasoned that I could use the exercise whether she was there or not - but the result is the same, I avoided using the phone.

Due to personal circumstances, she has had to deal with a lot of professionals - and has had to meet with panels of them on several occasions. The thought makes her ill – for weeks in advance – but she knows that she can go through with it. The thought makes my anxiety levels rise – yet she

ALL IN THE MIND

copes. She admits that it will seem surreal on the day – and she will not really be 'herself' – but she will come out, at the end of it, proud of herself.

I would say that Monica and Trudy share a slight aversion to the telephone too. They may make excuses, and have perfectly valid explanations as to why it is not really a problem for them, but this does not alter my opinion. They do not always answer the telephone. Monica has apologised for not answering my calls, explaining that she thought it might be someone else – and then she did not have enough credit to text me back. This may, of course, have been the case – but I know that she does not always feel like company and might be trying to save my feelings.

You see, although we all have problems, we are reluctant to actually admit it when we are going through a bad spell. It is much easier to talk about our quirks when we are 'ok' – we can dismiss our illogical actions for what they are from a comfortable distance – but it is very difficult to admit: 'Actually I'm not feeling too good at the moment and would rather be alone'. Admitting that you have a problem is just that – admitting that you have a problem – and no one wants to admit that they feel that they are weak or that they think that they are a failure.

Despite our sympathy for one another – and our inherent urge to comfort and protect one another – when we feel that we are unable to cope on an emotional level, the main feeling is that of embarrassment. We can logically state that we would hate for one of our friends to be ill and not feel that they could tell us – whilst feeling unable to confide in anyone when we feel ill ourselves.

It is this logical 'arguing back and forth' that is probably the most frustrating thing about the situation. When people – including professionals – try to talk you through the way you behave, getting you to acknowledge that it is illogical, it is really the last thing that you need. You are already aware that it is illogical – and to have that drummed into you again just makes you feel like even more of a failure.

The issue of driving actually causes problems for most of the people that I know – including myself. My sister experienced extreme anxiety before each driving lesson – and resorted to taking beta blockers for three days prior to sitting her test. She used to deal with this in the same way that she dealt with going out for a walk. She needed company. She wanted the moral support of a passenger – preferably someone who could drive – but as long as she did not have to face the journey alone she could cope.

To 'cope' is actually exaggerating her ability to drive. She was still ill before hand and her hands would visibly shake – but she managed to do what was necessary. Unfortunately she is no longer able to cope with these feelings of anxiety and avoids driving altogether – hoping that an emergency does

ALL IN THE MIND

not arise that would force her back into the driving seat.

Monica was unfortunate enough to suffer a panic attack at the wheel of her car. She now avoids driving too - but, admits that she has been able to drive, on the odd occasion, as long as she is alone – or her passenger is a non-driver.

I think these examples show that the root cause is much the same for both of them – perhaps they have a fear of failing or being seen as failures? One prefers to have someone there – ideally to take over if she finds herself unable to cope – whilst the other cannot cope with having her driving ability 'judged'. The main point is that they both hate driving and on the surface, this looks like the same problem – but how they feel and react to the problem is unique to *them*.

I am in a different position as I do not drive. I failed my test on several occasions - and the thought of getting behind the wheel now causes me to break out in a sweat! The traffic seems to be going at an alarming speed and I am terrified that I will not be quick enough to react. Confidence seems to be a contributory factor – and I have none where driving is concerned. But, as I failed my test this is not an issue. I do not have to make excuses not to drive – but I am glad that financially I have an excuse to postpone taking further lessons!

I would like to go back to the 'people phobia' mentioned earlier. As I have already stated I began to suspect I had problems, along this line, when I took to peeping through the curtains before going outside to hang out the washing. But I also experienced feelings of discomfort whilst taking and collecting my son from school. As I have already mentioned I do not drive, so we walked the mile, each way, in all winds and weather. The nearer I got to the school the more uncomfortable I would feel. It did not make any sense. I was not particularly friendly with the other mothers but I was not on bad terms with any of them either.

Now that the school 'run' has finished I find myself avoiding walking altogether. When I met Monica on the bus recently, she asked if I was on my way to work and I admitted that I was not – I was visiting my sister. She was appalled that I was taking the bus on such a short journey and implied that I was lazy. She tried to get me to accompany her to an aerobics class that evening, but the thought made me feel anxious – how could I possibly walk into a room full of people?

I was always considered quite shy but there came a time, especially after having children, that I became marginally more confident. I was still reasonably quiet but I could hold a conversation whilst waiting at the school gates. In fact, if someone looked lonely or anxious I could initiate the conversation. Being able to do so helped me to convince myself that I was 'ok'.

But as time went on I would dread seeing those little groups of people hovering outside the school

ALL IN THE MIND

gates. I am not comfortable in crowds and put my anxiety down to that – I could speak to individual people but the moment they congregated together I felt uneasy. I liked the other mothers - and would say 'Hello' in passing – but all together I viewed them as part of a group to which I did not belong.

What could I say that would interest or amuse them? In the end I would wait alone and probably managed to look quite aloof. It is easy to assume that someone who is quiet is perhaps 'snooty' or 'above themselves' but that may not be the case – they may feel trapped in a prison of their own making, unable to acknowledge that they have a problem, let alone be in a position to ask for help in dealing with it.

CHAPTER 4

Part of the reason that I decided to write this account was to try to understand my feelings and put them into words. The only person I discussed this project with was my sister - who has the uncomfortable ability to really make me acknowledge that I have a problem! She does not accept my denials and makes me explore the reasons for my actions – and she is the one with the most problems! It is true what they say: 'You cannot kid a kidder'. People with mental health problems can be pretty adept at recognizing them in other people.

She was already aware of the peg issue but, on reading my account of my laundry problems, it was a revelation to learn that I needed to hang out the washing in order of size. This made her admit to her need to hang out washing by the hem – trousers by their legs, tops upside down, etc. This is something that I need to do too but I had not recognized it as a problem.

I have tried to peg out the laundry in the order that it came out of the basket. I have tried to resist the urge to move the rest of the washing down the line - so that it can be hung out in its correct space – but it makes me feel anxious to leave it like that. Why? Again I do not know. Why do people avoid walking under ladders or say the phrase 'touch wood' if they feel that they are tempting fate? The truth is it moves you out of your 'comfort zone' and

ALL IN THE MIND

in order to regain that feeling of 'safeness' you need to obey the urge to do whatever it is that you are compelled to do.

I was about to ask my sister if she had ever tried to hang out her washing differently when she made an admission. She admitted that this 'quirk' forced her to go out into the garden and re-hang washing that her husband had pegged out 'incorrectly'.

So again we have this issue of feeling anxious if things are not done 'our' way. This made us come to an amazing realisation - this could possibly be a 'control' issue! It is true that our circumstances are different but, to varying degrees, we are both leading lives that are dictated by circumstance – therefore we are unable to make plans or promises because the situation could dictate that we have to cancel them.

Feeling that you are, at least, in control of hanging out the washing can give you a sense of comfort and satisfaction. But I am oversimplifying the situation here and would not like to suggest, for one moment, that this can explain every obsessive-compulsive action. The truth is I can only give an indication of how *I* feel about certain situations. I can only *imagine* how someone else feels - and any guess I make, in regards to the reason why, is just a theory. I do not have a medical background and I do not want to make any blanket generalizations.

I think that one of the main things that I have in common with my sister is that we think too much. We do not just accept things - we discuss them at length and try to analyze them. It is frustrating that with our combined knowledge and logic we are at a loss to explain why we react the way that we do!

For example we are both keen readers - I suppose it has been a means of escape since we were children. But my sister must dread reading on occasion, because once she starts a book she is compelled to read it through to the end – even if it is the most boring piece of rubbish that she has ever laid eyes upon!

She wishes that she did not have this compulsion – probably more than having to hang out the washing 'correctly' on the line – but she cannot stop herself. It is the same with magazines – she must start on page one and work her way through to the back page. She is not comfortable with picking out pages of interest.

I do not understand this compulsion myself – but I can relate to the feelings of anxiety that she feels if she does not stay in her 'comfort zone'. I suppose that is the point that I want to raise – whether you can understand someone's inability to cope with a situation or not, you should try to imagine how they feel. The reason that they feel anxious or afraid may be 'trivial' or 'bizarre' but the feelings will be anything but – those feelings are real.

ALL IN THE MIND

Tamsin cannot face the prospect of being in a social setting. People them selves can cause her anxiety but one of the main problems is her reluctance to use anyone else's cutlery, crockery and drinking vessels. It is not unusual, in the workplace, to put aside your own mug or cup but Tamsin has used her own mug at home for years. If it gets broken she cannot face using another one and a new one will need to be purchased. She also needs to use her own knife, fork and spoon as she cannot bear the thought of using cutlery that has been in someone else's mouth (however briefly). She used to visit a local public house, but the thought of using a glass that has touched someone else's lips, is no longer tolerable.

On the surface this appears to be a hygiene issue. But she denies that this is the case. She has always been uncomfortable in a social setting and maybe this is a side effect of that?

She is not comfortable using other people's cutlery and crockery so she avoids situations that will cause her to come into contact with that possibility. Maybe using her own 'property' acts like a security blanket? Maybe it is her way of remaining in her comfort zone?

Unfortunately I think that your 'comfort zone' can shrink. I find that I can no longer do things that, up until a year or so ago, I could do with relative ease. I went to college with my sister and continued to go when circumstances forced her to discontinue her studies. I resumed college a while later to study a different subject matter – but the thought of doing that now 'worries' me. I think that the less you do the more reluctant you become to do anything at all.

My sister was relieved when she was not forced to finish her formal school years in secondary school. But after a few years this relief changed to a sense of failure. She had hated school - and could never imagine a time when she would want to return to an educational establishment – but she regretted gaining no qualifications.

She was far from incapable – in fact, even though she missed a lot of school, they were unable to place her in a 'lower' stream when she actually went, as she was coping with the work that was set. But the fact that she had no formal qualifications made her *feel* incapable.

It is this sense of failure that she puts down to her inability to stop reading a book that she finds boring. To 'give up' re-establishes those feelings of being unable to see through. By reading it through to the end, she is satisfying herself that she can persevere and succeed at something. But this also highlights another issue. Despite going to college and gaining excellent grades in her qualifications, she still feels like a failure. Instead of concentrating on the certificates that she has gained, she dwells on her failure to finish school and her inability to complete her third year of college studies.

ALL IN THE MIND

Childhood seems to be the root cause of many problems. If you were a happy, popular child the chances are, you are a happy, popular adult. But if you were the unhappy loner – who always seemed to be either ignored or bullied – then those feelings of isolation and of 'not fitting in' will probably have intensified as you grew up.

I think I was reasonably happy in primary school. I was neither popular nor lonely – I seemed to be a typical child. I was one of a large family and never really gave a thought to an obvious lack of money. But I began to feel differently in secondary school.

I remember being on my way home from school one day, when one of my plimsolls fell out of my bag. For a moment I was tempted to pick it up – but then I noticed the large holes that were clearly visible in the soles, and changed my mind. Someone yelled 'Hey lost your dap?' and I lied and said that it wasn't mine - and it ended up being kicked around the road. I tried to find it funny and pretend that I was 'one of the crowd', but I do not think that I fooled anyone.

The emotions that I remember feeling on that occasion are still vivid. I was mortified and embarrassed. I wished that the ground could have opened up and swallowed me – and sometimes those feelings re-emerge when I least expect them. I feel out of my depth and as though I am trying to pretend that I am 'one of the crowd' – and everyone is increasingly aware that I am not.

These feelings are stronger when there are more people around. I arrive at work early so that I can avoid walking into a 'group' setting. The fewer people in a room, the more comfortable I feel. If more people arrive later I have at least established myself in that setting and it is less of an ordeal.

It is also the reason that I use the main entrance, at the front of the building, rather than go around to the side door - which leads into the room where all of my colleagues congregate before the workday commences. I would rather 'warn' them of my arrival – give them a chance to hear my key turning in the lock – than risk walking in on them. Perhaps walking in on them discussing me in an unsavoury way?

I guess this also highlights feelings of paranoia. But I have reserved that subject for another chapter.

ALL IN THE MIND

CHAPTER 5

Another side to these types of problems is depression. Knowing, or thinking, that you are unable to cope with certain situations can result in the decision to avoid any occasion that might cause you to feel anxious. You feel like a failure because you cannot cope, and this leads to feelings of inadequacy and depression. This can affect your ability to sleep and the type of dreams that you are likely to 'suffer'.

Joanne feels that she does not cope well at all and this is emphasized in her dreams. She has a recurrent dream in which she is in a car that is travelling down a very steep hill. By steep I mean virtually vertical. Everyone else on that road is happy and smiling. The sun is blazing, music is playing and she is the only one who appears to find the journey terrifying. She looks down and cannot imagine how the car is not toppling over but this does not appear to be bothering anyone else. This just makes her feel weak and vulnerable. Her waking feelings are being symbolized in a dream and she cannot escape the feelings of inadequacy and failure.

Georgina dreams of being unable to obtain a signal or response to her desperate efforts to phone someone. Either the phone will not ring, or she is cut off, or she is unable to hear the voice on the other end. Is this about feeling isolated? Or maybe it is symbolizing her belief that no one understands how she feels? It may even be that she feels she is unable to communicate with anyone?

Whatever the reason both dreamers wake feeling stressed and anxious and even more of a failure.

For Danielle it was not the dreams that bothered her but the sheer panic that she felt on waking one night. This was not like a panic attack but more of a distressing premonition of her impending death. She was absolutely certain that she was going to die and her main concern was who would take care of her children?

Like most mothers she had an overwhelming desire to protect her children and her impending death would mean that she would need to put certain safeguards in place. She was convinced that she would die before her husband returned from his nightshift, so she took the precaution of placing pillows and bedding around her bed in case her young baby fell and was hurt.

Some may believe that this 'premonition' had more to do with the fact that she was left alone, to care for her children, than anything else. A natural worry of what would happen in an emergency caused her to believe that she was going to face that emergency before daybreak.

In the same way as I took a solitary walk with my two young sons and ensured that we were armed with sticks, Danielle faced a solitary night and

ALL IN THE MIND

ensured that if the 'worst' happened her children would be safe.

But I have known of other people suffering these same feelings. Sophie too was convinced that she was going to die and it prevented her from making plans for the future. It also prevented her from reassuring her young son that she was not going to die. Sophie was not living on her own, nor left to take care of her children by herself, but she too was plagued by the 'premonition' that she was going to die. Why?

Is it the same worry that haunts every parent? Are we all programmed with the urge to protect our children, no matter what? Or is it because the birth of our children is a physical sign of our own mortality? The next generation is growing and developing so we are facing the realization that we are soon to become obsolete?

Is this why aging worries so many people? We are no longer the 'young ones' and must move aside for the next generation? Is this why we feel like failures? Like we are no longer useful members of society? Do we quantify age with importance? Some societies view their older generation as a 'font of wisdom and knowledge'. Maybe if we lived in another culture we would embrace aging in a more positive way.

If you feel old and worthless it can seem pointless to set a foot outside the front door. Age is not necessarily an indication of feeling old either.

Someone who is in their eighties or nineties can still have a positive outlook and enjoy a 'young' attitude, whilst others in their early thirties can appear to have lost all of their youth and vigour.

The problem is if you feel like this it is just another reason to avoid society. You cannot imagine anyone wanting to be in your company – or you fear that you will be unable to disguise how you feel – so you avoid going anywhere and then lose touch with people. The longer you stay out of contact, the more reluctant you become to get in touch - and the easier it becomes to avoid situations that may cause anxiety. But, the longer this goes on the more of a failure you feel and the more depressed you become. It is a vicious circle.

Of course depression affects people in as many different ways as the situations that cause anxiety and panic attacks. For some this means that they will avoid going out. Seeing other people looking happy and comfortable can make their feelings of inadequacy even more pronounced. For others, they may seem perfectly happy and comfortable, in a crowd of friends, but may be battling with feelings of depression just the same.

It all boils down to that 'comfort zone' again. Friends can have a cushioning effect and as long as a sufferer is in their presence they may feel more able to cope. Familiar places can have this effect too.

ALL IN THE MIND

Patricia is very reluctant to admit to her friends that she is uncomfortable in certain situations. She is able to cope if she knows the evening's plans, in advance, and no one defers from it but she needs to know how they are getting to and from a venue and the time-scales involved.

This all adds to cushion the affects of stepping outside of her 'comfort zone'. To most people she seems like the life and soul of the party - and if they later learn of her inability to hold down a job, through 'nerve' trouble, they may be forgiven for thinking that there is nothing wrong with her.

But this is a misconception. Just as my sister was unable to cope with school – but could go out with her friends in the evening – it did not make her feelings of anxiety and depression any less real. It is also what makes this illness all the more embarrassing and frustrating.

People who have never suffered with their 'nerves' have no idea how crippling it can be – and because no two people will be affected the same, it can cause doubt and confusion amongst acquaintances.

This can even be true among fellow sufferers. Just because *you* cannot deal with a situation does not mean that someone who *can,* is a 'fake'. They may very well feel that *you* are a fake because you are able to do things that they find impossible!

Another problem is that mental health issues can be genetic and therefore run in families. It is easy to dismiss a family as a group of 'skivers' just because none of them work - and they all seem to be doing 'very nicely' on benefits! But, as any doctor will tell you, if there are family members with a mental health issue it increases your chances of becoming a sufferer too.

Of course, the other side of the coin are the people who insist that they are unable to work, etc when there is nothing wrong with them. These people are probably one of the main reasons that a genuine sufferer feels embarrassed admitting to having problems in the first place!

There is a stigma attached to mental health issues. Unless you are unfortunate enough to be very obviously affected, there are generally no outward signs of your illness – especially if you are adept at avoiding situations that cause you problems.

It is a little like that old medical chestnut 'the bad back'. There are many genuine sufferers who will know how debilitating this can be – but there is very little medical proof, sometimes, to back up the symptoms. Therefore a genuine sufferer will be in pain and feel frustrated – but may be reluctant to admit to suffering from a bad back because they might be met with a knowing smile or a dubious 'I see'.

ALL IN THE MIND

Sufferers may then become depressed and anxious about going out, because they do not want to answer awkward questions and be made to feel like they are a liar or are simply too lazy to work. Meanwhile the person using the 'bad back' excuse – specifically because it is not always easy to diagnose – will have no problem relating this to every Tom, Dick and Harry. And this increases the feelings of embarrassment and frustration in a genuine sufferer. But this does not mean that anyone who admits to a bad back is a liar – it just makes him or her feel like one!

If there was a test that the medical profession could carry out, to determine how 'bad' your nerves are, I have no doubt that every genuine sufferer would volunteer to have it performed tomorrow – providing that it was a good day and they were capable of visiting the surgery!.

Being prescribed medication can be an indication – but I know a few people who have 'borrowed' symptoms from genuine sufferers that they know, and have been prescribed anti-depressants on the strength of what they 'say' is wrong with them.

Unfortunately there are always going to be people who will abuse the system and give genuine sufferers a bad name – and this, added to the fact that society is not always as compassionate as it could be, just confirms the public consensus that sufferers are a 'load of layabouts'!

I suppose that the main purpose of writing this is to raise awareness of just how difficult it is to admit to having a mental health problem. If someone makes this kind of admission it should be met with empathy and compassion – and the realisation that it took a lot of courage for them to speak out. The main feeling to avoid is pity. No one requires 'tea and sympathy' at this crucial moment. They just need understanding. Actually, I am making a blanket generalization – something that I generally try to avoid but am still guilty of doing on a regular basis!

I suppose everyone will need different things from different people. Tea and sympathy may well hold a place for some people, in the process of coming to terms with admitting that there is a problem – it just might not be right for *all* sufferers.

There is probably only one hard and fast rule and that is that there *are* no hard and fast rules! Each person is an individual and is going to need to approach their problems in their own way. I would say that the most important thing that you can offer is your support.

You can admit to a total lack of understanding. In fact encouraging a sufferer to explain how they feel (even if they are unable to explain why) may prove very beneficial for all concerned – but if you make it clear that you are there for them (on their terms) it can do nothing but good. One thing to be aware of though, is that it may highlight a few problems of your own – a few little quirks that you like to dismiss

ALL IN THE MIND

as nothing. But, I wonder if you will be brave enough to admit that *you* have a problem?

CHAPTER 6

Dealing with anxiety, panic attacks and depression are, again, as varied as the symptoms experienced by different sufferers. Some people assume that the doctor will think it is a 'trivial' problem and dismiss them with the phrase 'pull yourself together'! I would like to assure those people that there are very few doctors today who will view their problems in that way. Most agree that a patient's mental health is just as important as their physical well being.

Other people, however, will go to the doctor's surgery as their first 'port of call'. They will discuss their feelings and agree upon a course of action with their physician. It does not mean that they are less or more affected than the former – they are just able to deal with their problems differently.

But for some people, a visit to see the doctor can be a daunting prospect. They may not feel able to cope with the act of physically walking into the surgery – let alone admitting to the doctor that they think that they are 'going mad'!

How do you get the help that you need if you are unable to ask for it? If you are able to walk into the surgery and make an appointment, you are half way there. But if you feel unable to broach the subject maybe writing down your thoughts and feelings will help.

ALL IN THE MIND

This is the course of action that my sister takes – and the action that I have taken in the past. It negates the need to speak, unless the doctor needs to ask any questions, and it can also help alleviate the concern that you will cry. It probably will not prevent the tears – feeling like a failure tends to upset most people – but it will make it easier for the doctor to understand the situation, should tears ensue.

But what if you are unable to walk into the surgery? If you do not have an aversion to the telephone then you can simply pick up the receiver and dial – but I have been in the position of being unable to take either course of action! Generally you are faced with a choice. Wait until you feel more able to cope – not every sufferer will feel at their lowest ebb all of the time – or enlist the help of someone else. Unfortunately, neither is absolutely guaranteed to succeed. You may feel that you are never going to feel any better, or feel unable to confess your feelings to anyone else.

Once that initial hurdle is overcome, and the doctor has an indication of how you feel, then the treatment is discussed. Is the cause of the problem situational? Does your life, where you live, your neighbours, etc have an impact on how you feel? Or is it less identifiable than that?

For some people, talking through their anxieties with a psychologist, psychiatrist or counsellor will be the preferred option. For others, medication may be prescribed as a temporary measure. For yet others, stronger medication – mood stabilizers, anti psychotic drugs, etc - may need to be used on a more permanent basis.

The trouble with drugs is that if they work – and you feel better – there is a tendency to stop taking them because you believe that you are 'cured'. When the feelings re-emerge it can make you feel even worse than before. Another problem is the stress that you are under when you are faced with these difficulties. Stress again affects people differently. Some people thrive on it – whilst others buckle under the weight of it.

But stress can be the root cause of many physical problems. I find my concentration and memory are affected when I feel stressed. I will decide to check that the backdoor is locked before going out, and then realise that I probably left the bathroom light on. I will go upstairs to check (turning off any lights that have been inadvertently left on) and then return downstairs. I am then not sure if I checked the backdoor before going upstairs or, if I was waylaid on my way to the backdoor, so I check the backdoor again. This is because my concentration is not what it should be because I am stressed – and, to make matters worse, I cannot trust my memory either!

I do not check and recheck it on purpose. I do not have an obsession about it – in fact if I am going to the local shop I will not bother locking the door at all. But, because I am not fully concentrating on the

ALL IN THE MIND

task the first time, I am aware that I do repeat it 'just to be sure'.

I do the same thing with the kitchen tap. When you turn it on it flows really well – but the power reduces and it becomes a trickle. You tend to have to turn it again so that full power resumes. Or this was the case up until I thought 'I'll just do that for a minute whilst the sink is filling up' – and then wondered what the noise of rushing water was! The water had lost none of its power and had filled the sink and was cascading over the sides onto the floor! I now check the tap – and then check it again – and then check it again, before leaving the room, 'just to be sure'.

I believe that is where most of these things start to have a hold over you. You return home to find a door which you are sure that you locked, open. You are concerned because you realise that it is not safe to do so in this day and age – but confused too. Then you do not trust yourself. 'Did I lock that door?' 'Did I turn off that tap?' – and you find yourself double checking 'just to be sure'.

It then becomes like a talisman or 'security blanket'. To check things, and double check things, are another way of staying in your 'comfort zone'. It reassures you and makes you feel safe.

If you are forced to interrupt this 'checking' ritual it can leave you feeling anxious and afraid, and that awful feeling of 'impending doom' hits you. If you do not check that door at least 10 times you cannot feel certain that it is locked – someone could break in whilst you are out, and you will never feel safe again.

Kate has been diagnosed as being 'bi polar'. She cleans religiously and bleaches everything to within an inch of its life when she is stressed. Her hands become red and inflamed (because she 'forgets' to wear rubber gloves) and it makes her physically ill. But mentally she 'needs' to do this. In order to feel safe, and keep her anxiety levels at bay, she 'needs' to go through this process even though she knows that she is making herself ill.

She has manic moments when she is full of energy and has an enthusiasm for life – at times like this she can be exhausting to be around. Unfortunately these are balanced with feelings of despair. She has no energy and cannot see the point in anything. She goes from being a bubbly person to someone who is withdrawn, tearful and lethargic. She is unable to concentrate, when low, and her memory is poor. She is reluctant to bathe or shower – despite having a high level of personal hygiene at other times – and cannot be bothered to do anything. Even for other people.

I suppose this is another aspect of mental illness. At times it can almost be regarded as selfish. You become very wrapped up in how awful you feel and are unable to raise an interest in other people's lives. This implies that you do not care. But, on some levels, I think it is because you care too much. Other people's problems can sometimes

ALL IN THE MIND

drag you down until you feel so low yourself that you are simply not able to cope with anything else.

I often tell people that they need to look after themselves first. If they do not look after themselves they are not going to be capable of looking after anyone else. I think that when people hit a 'low spot' it is their brain's way of saying 'enough'. It needs to shut down and recharge.

It is sometimes because we think too much about how other people feel or think, that we make ourselves ill worrying about it. I personally believe that if people could force themselves to be a little more 'selfish' in the first place, they may avoid a lot of the guilt brought about by depression and anxiety.

CHAPTER 7

Sometimes it can be easy to find an excuse for behaviour that deviates from the 'norm'. A couple that I know has had the misfortune to be involved in several car accidents during recent years. The wife Nora does not drive herself so she can in no way be held accountable for those accidents. Nor can her husband Arthur, who was the driver in at least two of them, - as they were shown to be the fault of a third party – but it has had a impact on both on them.

Arthur is now a nervous driver and this is made worse by the fact that his wife is a nervous passenger – so much so that she has taken to travelling in the back of the car! She feels less inclined to comment on how close they seem to be to other cars and he is less inclined to shout at her for accusing him of driving too close!

Nora no longer has any confidence travelling by car – and this is obvious in the way that she holds on to the hand strap above the passenger door! She realises that her behaviour has a direct impact on her husband's confidence in his ability to drive but she cannot help it.

I too am a nervous passenger. My husband would call that an understatement! I regularly accuse him of speeding and driving too close to the car in front. I also gasp and close my eyes when he takes, what looks to me, like 'stupid risks' on a

ALL IN THE MIND

roundabout. He regularly shouts at me and reminds me that I can't even drive – but that is irrelevant. I do not wish to drive but it does not stop me from ramming my foot down on a non-existent brake!

Maybe it is that control element again? From that point of view I feel entirely at his mercy – I am zooming around amongst traffic that looks like a blur and he appears to be pulling out into a roundabout, when there does not seem to be a gap!

I have noticed something in the above paragraph that hits the nail on the head. 'Zooming around *amongst* traffic' – I do not feel like a *part* of that traffic. The traffic is something that is going on around me – I guess that could be a metaphor for life. I could blame my detachment to the rest of the traffic on my inability to drive – but I do not think that would be a true assessment of the situation.

Being behind the wheel of a car does not make me feel any more a part of the traffic than being in the passenger seat. I do not really see that having a steering wheel in front of you means that you are in control of that vehicle. Too many things can go wrong. You do not have to worry about only *your* driving – you have to worry about everyone else's too!

My eldest son recently yelled at me for panicking when his father was approaching a roundabout. He said that I was going to cause him to have an accident if I kept on like that! He could not believe I could be that nervous a passenger! As far as I was concerned my behaviour was perfectly reasonable – I could not understand how my son felt safe – but I suppose he was looking at things from another angle. He knows that his father would not endanger our lives and felt that my attitude was the problem. But, knowing that is not going to make travelling with my husband any less traumatic in the future!

It is not just my husband's driving that I find difficult to cope with – although I do find it more difficult travelling with him than with anyone else - I find buses a problem too. With buses though, it is not just the driving that bothers me – it is the people on the bus. The more people on the bus the more anxious I become.

I have always been annoyed with people sitting in the front seats when they are perfectly capable of walking further up the bus – but I find myself doing this myself. Ironically, if the bus is empty, I have no problem walking to the back of the bus – but, the fuller the bus, the more inclined I am to sit near the front. I use the excuse that at least I am willing to give up my seat for someone less able to stand – and this is true – but it is mainly because I cannot face walking past a lot of people to reach a vacant seat.

Here we are back to 'people' again. But, some people are easier to cope with than others. I watch GMTV every morning and enjoy the light-hearted

ALL IN THE MIND

way in which they deal with the news items. I generally find the news depressing and avoid it when at all possible as it tends to play on my mind, but I find 'Good Morning Television' very easy to watch.

But there is always one bit that I find difficult to watch – Keith Chegwin arriving, unannounced, at someone's home first thing in the morning! The fact that he is delivering a cheque for ten thousand pounds is totally lost on me – it could be ten million pounds and I still would not like to find him at my door! That is never going to be a problem that I will have to face, as I can never bring myself to enter those competitions. I do not find Tony Blackburn such a problem but then he does not threaten to turn up on my doorstep!

Please do not misunderstand me - I do not actually dislike Keith Chegwin. I think it has more to do with him being so spontaneous. No one ever seems to know what he will do next and I find that very disconcerting!

You would be forgiven for thinking that my acquaintances must be a miserable bunch. But, ironically, we all share the ability to laugh at our misfortunes. We all have a pretty good sense of humour and are able to see the funny side of most situations. Unfortunately this also extends to laughing at other people's misfortunes too!

I think that the tendency to laugh at 'inappropriate' times is, in itself, a form of nerve trouble - or it could simply be your brain's way of coping with stress. If someone tells you "There's so and so over there – don't look", the urge to look becomes overwhelming. In much the same way as being told not to think of a pink elephant will make it almost impossible to think of anything else!

The moment that I know it is inappropriate to laugh, the more difficult it seems to be to fight the urge. What is worse is that anyone who knows me will immediately look at me to see if I have managed to quell it! This can be embarrassing and annoying – not to mention downright rude – but if you find yourself in this situation it can be very difficult to explain.

My sister and I often think that our troubles could be the basis for a very funny 'situation comedy'. She insists that our inability to drive, cope with different people and situations would appeal to a lot of people – and there lies a ray of sunshine in an otherwise cloudy sky. We can see the absurdity of our reactions but can, when the chips are down, see the funny side.

We imagine that the central characters – ourselves – have somehow gotten themselves into working for a delivery firm. We both hate driving so this raises a smile – not to mention our anxiety levels! Neither of us are very good map-readers and we have an aversion to talking to strangers – so our characters would get lost and be unable to ask for directions! Then, to put the tin hat on it, both would be suggesting that the other one calls the

ALL IN THE MIND

office for assistance because neither wants to use the phone!

Having a sense of humour is pretty much essential to coping sometimes. It does not help the situation but it does alleviate the build up of emotions as an alternative to crying. Of course it can be met with as much confusion, and sometimes with looks of disapproval, but laughter is the body's own stress reliever. It takes far fewer muscles to smile than to frown.

CHAPTER 8

In the previous chapter I mentioned having an inappropriate sense of humour - and how other people can view this embarrassing habit of laughing at the wrong moment. I have also mentioned being compelled to carry out certain tasks in an almost ritualistic manner, the fact that I dislike change and that I am uncomfortable when having to step outside of my 'comfort zone'.

Looking at these 'symptoms' on their own – having an inappropriate sense of humour, liking a set routine/disliking change, being comfortable in a familiar setting and perhaps becoming 'obsessive' about certain things, you could be forgiven for thinking that there are similarities with autism.

I was struck by these similarities when visiting an acquaintance, Claudia recently and the subject of Liam came up. Liam is 6 years old and a typically boisterous little boy – but he is unable to sit quietly, cannot cope in a crowded or noisy place and is unable to concentrate on more than one thing at a time.
He has been diagnosed as having Asperger's Syndrome which affects those at the higher end of the autistic spectrum. Sufferers at this end can sometimes be regarded as gifted but it would be a misconception to assume that all of those with Asperger's Syndrome, will be near geniuses.

ALL IN THE MIND

Asperger's syndrome is a type of autism and it is quite clear that those with autism do not cope very well with change – but neither do many people suffering with mental health issues. Could some autistic traits then be linked to the more common mental health disorders?

Liam also develops obsessions with certain items as well as feeling compelled to carry out certain tasks. He went through a vigorous hand-washing phase but his main concern was ensuring that the soap was on the 'correct' side of the hand basin. If it was placed on the other side he was 'compelled' to move it and became quite anxious if he was asked to leave it where it was.

If an adult behaved in this way they would be regarded as suffering from an 'obsessive compulsive' disorder – I am not aware of any adults who feel compelled to do this type of thing, that have been diagnosed with autism. This begged the question why would a six year old be diagnosed with Asperger's Syndrome when an adult would be regarded as having developed an obsessive/compulsive disorder?

One of Liam's older relatives, Oliver, has a few obsessions of his own – mainly needing to stick to certain routines which cause him anxiety if they are disturbed. Could Liam have picked up on these 'rituals' and then developed a few of his own? Or is it merely because they are relatives and therefore share the same genes?

It has been previously stated that mental health issues tend to run in families – but is this merely because a young child is 'learning' to develop these traits, or does the fact that they share the same genes have a bearing on whether or not a mental health issue will erupt?

It is that age-old question on what affects us most: 'Nature or nurture'? Are we born pre-ordained to develop certain things in a certain way, or does the way in which we are 'nurtured' play a part?

If Liam and an adult with similar 'symptoms' visit a specialist, will they be given the same diagnosis? Will the adult be diagnosed with Asperger's Syndrome or be told that they have an obsessive/compulsive disorder? Will the child be told that they are 'too young' to have 'bad nerves', or to develop this sort of disorder, and be given a different diagnosis to the adult? And would this simply be because of the difference in their ages rather than their 'symptoms'?

Obviously I have no medical background and what appears to me to be the 'same' thing may, in fact, be entirely different. But, I find the similarities interesting just the same.

Anyone with a mental health issue will be able to understand Liam's inability to sit still. I find that I am unable to sit still when using the telephone at home. This could be because even when I am able to use it I am not 'comfortable' and pacing back and

ALL IN THE MIND

forth is a way of coping with these feelings of unease. I also find myself pacing back and forth whilst waiting for the bus. In cold weather this can be explained by a desire to keep warm but on a hot summer's day that excuse does not sound very plausible.

When you are anxious it is difficult to sit or stand still. Think of a time when you were waiting for something, when you were *anxiously* waiting for something – to leave for an appointment, a date, or a driving lesson perhaps, or for the arrival of a family member, or for news of how you did in your examinations – were you able to sit quietly and read a magazine or watch television?

When you are anxious your ability to concentrate is diminished and doing anything 'constructive' becomes increasingly difficult. You can attempt to read a magazine article or complete a crossword puzzle, but the worry that is causing your anxiety will seep into your consciousness until you have to give up.

Pacing and rocking back and forth are a kind of 'comfort'. Maybe these stem back from being rocked in your mother's arms or when she paced up and down in an effort to 'settle' you – whatever the reason, rocking and pacing are an indication of deep rooted anxiety. That said, I often rock from side to side but this is a bi-product of nursing my children – you can recognize the difference because your stance indicates the absence of a baby!

Anyone suffering with agoraphobia will associate with Liam's reluctance to be in a crowded and noisy place. In fact this reluctance is quite common in children and you only have to kneel down, to their level, to see why. Crowds are not pleasant – especially when viewed at a height that puts you at the disadvantage of not being able to see above anyone else's head. But those with autism are said to see crowds from a different angle again.

Those that suffer with, what has been termed 'noise and visual' intolerance are said to see a crowded shopping centre as 'speeded up'. Have you ever fast forwarded a film and tried to select the scene for which you are looking? It is difficult to make sense of it and after a while you have to press the 'Play' button to ease the chaos in front of your eyes. Unfortunately those with 'visual' intolerance are unable to press the play button and are bombarded with images that they cannot make sense of. Is it any wonder that they drop to the floor, scream, and cry, and refuse to walk further?

Noise intolerance is self explanatory – yet what can seem a 'comfortable' volume, for the majority of people, can have a sufferer clutching painfully at his ears in an effort to block out the intrusion on his eardrums.

Discos, parties and raves are havens for flashing lights and a cacophony of different sounds – so maybe a reveler would have difficulty in comprehending the problem. But imagine how you feel the morning after - and then imagine having to

ALL IN THE MIND

contend with the rumble of a jackhammer outside of your bedroom window. Not a pleasant thought is it?

CHAPTER 9

I touched on the subject of paranoia at the end of an earlier chapter. This has probably affected us all at some point in our lives. It is that awful feeling when you walk into a room and the conversation suddenly stops. Or the look that you get when you walk past people that you know vaguely, but with whom you are not really on very good terms.

I am generally philosophical about it – when they are talking about me they are giving someone else a rest – but it is not a pleasant feeling nonetheless. The trouble is we all enjoy a bit of harmless gossip – providing that we are not too closely connected to it, of course - because it is not very enjoyable when you are the subject of the local grapevine banter.

But what if those feelings become apparent for no reason? You could walk past people having a totally innocent conversation, and then misread a look or phrase and simply jump to conclusions. That is not a problem in itself – if you are the type of person who can walk away from such a situation – but what if you then demand to know what the problem is? The situation can then escalate out of control. You will think you have every right to know what is being said about you and to justify yourself – whereas the other people may not want to tell you what they were saying and refuse to discuss it further.

ALL IN THE MIND

The sad thing is that if they were to try to convince you that they were not talking about you, they would be unable to do so. Their denials would just infuriate you even more – not only did they have the nerve to talk about you they were then too much of a coward to admit it and had now resorted to lying! A bad situation then gets even worse because after accusing totally innocent people of talking about you, you now become the topic of their conversation! Now, to the person unaffected by feelings of paranoia this may sound a little bizarre – but just think how it feels to actually be in that situation?

Many women go through the menopause with ease. For some, however, the transition is not quite so uneventful. Whilst some women merely suffer 'hot flushes' and restlessness, others can develop depression and mood swings. For the unfortunate few, things can escalate beyond even that.

Dianne experienced feelings of paranoia that really made her think that not only was she going mad but that her family was trying to drive her there! She accused them of moving objects and hiding things. As much as they tried to convince her otherwise she was absolutely sure that they were guilty! Things came to a crux when she accused them of hiding a dishcloth! After being placed on appropriate medication she began to improve and could see for herself how 'ridiculous' her claims had been – but whilst being ill they had made total sense to her.

She can laugh about it now but imagine how frightened she must have been? She thought that her family was trying to drive her insane and was aware that no one believed her. It did not make any difference how many people tried to convince her that it was 'all in her mind' – to her it was real.

Many people suffer tinnitus – or noises in the ear. It is easy for a non-sufferer to tell the person that it is 'all in the mind' but that is of no help to the sufferer. Imagine a jackhammer digging up the road outside your window. You can hear it, you can feel those vibrations and the stress it puts you under almost causes you to go outside and throw that jackhammer down the nearest manhole! Now, imagine that you look outside but there is no jackhammer. You can hear it, you can feel those vibrations and your stress levels are rising through the roof – but you cannot see it. Complaining to your family results in confused looks and raised eyebrows, whilst a visit to the doctor would probably confirm tinnitus.

Now the fact that you have been made aware that the noise is not real is not going to make it any easier to deal with, is it? In fact the realisation that it is 'all in the mind' is probably the catalyst that you do not need.

Have you ever had a lucid dream? Those are the kind that you have when you know that you are dreaming. What about the other sort of dream? The ones where really bizarre things happen but they seem absolutely true? Well I suppose it must

ALL IN THE MIND

be a little like that. When you wake up you realise that it was a dream – and of course it was a dream! How could you ever have thought that it could really happen? But, until you wake up, you are stuck believing something is true even though it is not possible - and other people can only view it as bizarre!

Of course there is another side to this coin. Sometimes you can be doubtful something is happening, when it is, because you no longer trust yourself to draw the correct conclusion.

Gaynor was certain that the half term holidays were over a week away but, when an acquaintance convinced her that they began at the end of the current week, she was doubtful at first, but then accepted this as fact when faced with such a positive affirmation. If she had trusted her own judgement more, she would have perhaps been able to point out logically why she was sure that the acquaintance was wrong. But a few positive statements to the contrary convinced her that *she* was wrong – even though a quick glance at the calendar back at home proved that she was right.

The point is that if something is 'all in the mind' it is in the very place where it can do the most damage. Your mind can play tricks on you and make you see and hear things that are not real – or vice versa - and you may find yourself incapable of distinguishing between fantasy and reality.

CHAPTER 10

Confidence is a factor in how you view yourself and how others perceive you. It is no coincidence then that the profession that attracts the most insecure people in the world is also 'home' to a host of mental health problems.

I am, of course, talking about the 'fame' industry in all its guises. Stephen Fry has recently completed a documentary on his life as a BI-polar sufferer. He enlisted the help and support of other celebrities – including Robbie Williams – to highlight the illness and help lift the veil – if not the stigma – on mental health problems.

Performers typify my theory that people are able to put on a 'public' face and give an outward appearance of calm even though they are suffering inside. To a certain extent they also help to show the degree to which a person can suffer before their 'mask' slips.

Stephen Fry famously walked out of a theatre performance and disappeared for several days because he was unable to cope with the pressure. But was it the pressure to perform on stage that got to him, or was it the pressure to pretend to be something that he was not?

We all have an image of ourselves that we want to project – and to a certain degree we all 'pretend' to be something other than we are. We do not want

ALL IN THE MIND

our children to view us as stupid or afraid and so we may feel able to do more, on their behalf, than we would otherwise attempt. We also have a desire to protect and comfort them so we are capable of pushing ourselves a little further outside of our 'comfort zone' for them.

But if you have done that then you will know how exhausting and stressful it can be. To push yourself a 'little further' can be a rewarding experience – but it can also be a terrifying one. So if someone in the public eye is constantly trying to push themselves a 'little further' it is not so difficult to see why they should, eventually, 'burn themselves out', is it?

Performers are renowned for suffering stage fright and feeling ill before going out on to the stage. So why do they do it? Why do they push themselves out of their comfort zone? How are they able to cope with that amount of pressure? Maybe the validation that they get from audience approval is more rewarding than the fear gripping them before they step out in front of the footlights?

Robbie Williams stated that he could perform in front of thousands of people and then go to his trailer and hide under the bedcovers. Why? What makes a man, who can be such a lively entertainer, want to hide away? Maybe he finds it exhausting to wear his public mask for more than a couple of hours. Maybe the pressure to feel that he has to 'put on a show', gets too much for him and he needs to 'be himself'. Therefore the mask slips and he becomes afraid of how others will perceive him and so he has to hide himself away.

It may simply be that he cannot face people as himself, and so when he has finished performing, his brain shuts down and he needs to recharge his batteries. The pressure that he puts on himself is simply not sustainable.
Of course I am only guessing; the only person who really knows how he feels is Robbie Williams, himself.

The thought of stepping out onto a stage is too terrifying for me to comprehend – I cannot understand what could possess someone to do it. But then I feel much the same way at the thought of leaping from a plane! The truth is some people enjoy the adrenaline rush. They like to push past that sense of fear. Robbie Williams and Stephen Fry may be 'adrenaline junkies' – pushing themselves to 'jump out of the plane' but, on landing, feel that they need to recuperate for a while. Only the plane is a stage and to recuperate they need to hide away. Who knows?

Stephen Fry enjoys his manic episodes – as do most Bi-polar sufferers – and feels that they contribute to his creativity. In this 'hyped up' state he feels indestructible and capable of doing anything; so much so that he avoids medication because he fears that it will hamper his imagination and make him less 'himself'.

ALL IN THE MIND

Others are not so convinced that these 'highs' are worth the extreme dips that plunge them into despair. At low points they are all-consumed with thoughts of suicide and cannot be comforted – it is this aspect that is frightening, because they find it almost impossible to claw themselves out of this chasm. Unfortunately many sufferers do give in to the urge to 'end it all'.

It has been pointed out to me that they might not actually want to die but cannot see another way of stopping what is going on in their lives. They want to 'end it all' but not in the sense that they want to die. They just may not be able to think of another way of escaping their problems or the feelings that plague them.

Obviously, at this end of the scale, medication is vital to stabilise the mood swings and to keep things on a more or less even keel. Ironically sufferers at this end are more likely to stop their medication during 'good' spells because they will not only feel 'cured' but indestructible too! Either end of the spectrum can be dangerous because risks are taken during 'good' spells – when sufferers feel that they can do anything – and during 'bad' spells when they simply do not care.

Of course, confidence – or a lack of it – does not only affect the famous. Hailey is a tall lady and has a larger than life personality. Her vibrant hair colour is a real head turner – so it seemed quite bizarre to realise that she was shy. Instead of hiding away – which would have been quite impossible anyway -

she chose to draw attention to herself. You may ask yourself why, but this is a trick we have all done on occasion. By 'pretending' to be confident and having a 'hey look at me!' attitude she actually avoided unwanted attention. If you saw a large lady with vibrant hair, would you want to hassle her?

It is the same thing that crime prevention experts suggest. It does not take a genius to work out that a mugger is far more likely to attack a small, quiet, victim – someone who looks weak and vulnerable – than a large, confident looking individual, does it?

By dressing confidently, and behaving in a way that suggests that we are perfectly comfortable with the situation, we are almost able to convince ourselves that everything is ok. And we, more than anyone else, are harder to kid because we know what frightens us most. If we can convince ourselves ensuring that other people believe our 'act', is a piece of cake!

But what if we cannot convince ourselves that everything is ok? What if the self-doubt and feelings of inadequacy are all consuming? How can you cope then? Well, that is when you end up going through a bad spell and there is very little that you can do about it. Not a very encouraging thought maybe, but an honest one. It is like someone losing a loved one and being told that they must 'pull themselves together'.

When you feel that your life is falling apart, and you really begin to think that you would be better off

ALL IN THE MIND

dead, then it is going to take a little more than a 'pull yourself together' to get you into a more positive frame of mind! Sometimes it is simply better to ride out the storm. Medication may help – mood stabilisers, if you have been prescribed them – but for some the help that they need may simply be time. Very rarely is a bad spell going to be long term – if you seem unable to see the light at the end of the tunnel then obviously more intense help is required.

It helps to remind yourself that the bad feelings will not last. But recognising that, when you feel as though things are never going to get any better, is difficult to say at the least. Maybe writing down positive thoughts, when you are going through a good spell, will help? But the problem is that what can seem logical and straightforward when you are well, can make you feel as though you are wading through treacle when you are ill. What seemed like a good idea appears ludicrous and pointless. When you are arguing with your rational self there seems very little hope does there?

CHAPTER 11

I have already mentioned that my sister's inability to speak to people resulted in her being regarded as 'snooty'- and this raises an interesting point. Because people behave in a way that it is not easily understood, it is easy to misinterpret their actions.

Helen is a young, single mother who lives a considerable distance from her family. When she visited a distant relative she struck up a conversation with the daughter of the house, Rose, who, seeing how much Helen's child enjoyed the company of her own children, assured her that she was welcome at anytime – just phone first to ensure that she was in.

A few days later Helen phoned and asked if it was ok to visit and was assured that it was – she then asked Rose if she would come and collect her and then drive her back home later. Now Rose, who was due to go to work later, did not have the time to play taxi driver and explained that although she was happy for Helen to visit she would need to make her own way there and back – Helen made her excuses and postponed her visit.

To some people, Helen expecting Rose – whom she did not know very well – to make four car trips (collecting Helen, driving her to her home, taking her back home later and then drive home herself) is a little 'cheeky'. But, when you realise that Helen is 'uncomfortable' travelling on her own, you realise

ALL IN THE MIND

that things are not quite as cut and dried, as they seemed. You may not view Helen's request as the least bit cheeky – in a society that sees children being driven here, there and everywhere - asking for a 'lift' is hardly the faux pas of the century is it?

But this raises another point. Our upbringing tends to dictate how we view things. The majority of my own family was brought up to believe that asking for anything was wrong. So asking for a 'lift' is viewed upon as being 'cheeky'. You waited to be offered and even then you refused, out of politeness, because you did not want to 'put someone out' or be a bother to them.

Others are brought up with the motto 'if you do not ask you do not get'. Why not ask for a lift? If it is not convenient your request will be refused and if you are offering to pay for the 'privilege' what is the problem? This of course proves the fact that your childhood and upbringing can have a longstanding effect on the rest of your life.

We were brought up with the knowledge that we did not have a lot of money and that we were never to ask for anything. It was drummed into us from any early age, that if our mother could afford to buy us something then she would do so. If she did not buy it then it was because she did not have any spare money to spend and we must not embarrass her by asking.

I remember when Christmas was approaching my sister and I would be asked to look through the catalogue to choose something. But we never chose what we really wanted because we were very conscious of the fact that money was 'tight'. We would look for cheaper items and try to pretend that we were not disappointed. The meaning of Christmas was not lost on us either. We were always reminded that it was not just about presents – so, the fact that we would not be receiving the latest Barbie or Pippa doll was hardly the end of the world.

It was important that we were seen as 'good' and 'kind'. We were brought up to believe that you should always put other people first and to consider their feelings. These are important lessons, and I am not trying to diminish them in any way, but I believe that there is a limit to the expectations that you should put on other people.

Sometimes, it is not other people's expectations but our own that is the problem. Being nice, kind and polite are all good qualities that we would like to nurture in others and ourselves. Being polite seems a little old fashioned today when respect seems to be a thing of the past, but I was brought up to think that this was extremely important. Politeness seems to go hand in hand with punctuality. It is not polite to keep people waiting. But sometimes that is unavoidable.

As I have mentioned previously, I do not drive so I rely on public transport. As a rule I find it pretty good – although I have been known to say 'buses always run late except when *you* are!' If I have to

ALL IN THE MIND

be somewhere I catch an earlier bus than necessary 'just to be on the safe side'. But sometimes even that precaution is fruitless when two buses or more fail to turn up!

That happened recently when I was visiting my sister and I found myself getting a shade anxious. I did not feel able to use my mobile telephone so was unable to let her know that I was running late. I was stuck waiting at a bus stop until the next bus turned up. When my sister and I discussed this she admitted that she felt anxious if they were caught in traffic, on their way to collect their son from school. Actually anxious is an understatement – the word she used was 'frantic'. If her husband could telephone and warn them of the delay, then this eased her 'anxiety' a little but it did not stop it altogether.

We both felt that this was due to our unwillingness to let people down. When we are expected somewhere we like to be there not just on time but early. If anyone is going to be kept waiting then let it be us! It is a wonderful idea to put other people first and to always consider how other people feel. If everyone did that then we would all be happy and feel cared for – but if everyone else is 'looking after number one' then who is going to put *you* first? We are back at the 'selfish' point again but I feel it is a point worth reiterating.

Pam is a placid, easy-going woman who will do anything for a quiet life. She does not want to 'rock the boat' and allows the general day to day niggles of married life pass her by. So what if her husband drinks a little too much and he and the kids take her for granted? Life is too short to make a fuss, isn't it? But, the problem is those little 'niggles' add up and then something trivial happens and she blows! Her family thinks that she is potty. What is her problem? Nothing in her life has changed so why is she suddenly making a fuss?

The point is that it was not the trivial event that caused Pam to lose her temper. That trivial thing had just been added to every other little incident that she has simply 'let go' over the past few weeks or months. She has spent so long trying to put things to the back of her mind that there is simply no room left there for it.

The problem is that when you put things to the back of your mind that is where they stay – in your mind. That is where they fester and grow and cause physical problems. It is much healthier to voice an opinion and to tell someone how unhappy their actions are making you. But this is difficult if you have been brought up to believe that you have no right to put your feelings at the top of your list.

If you do not look after yourself how will you be able to look after someone else? It is not selfish to put your own needs and desires on a parallel with other peoples' – in fact I would say that it is crucial to do so. Recognising your own worth goes a long way to helping you realise that you are a relevant human being and just as important as anyone else.

ALL IN THE MIND

CHAPTER 12

Writing this has made me examine my past more closely in order to try to determine when, exactly, my problems started. It is easy to think of an event that made me feel uncomfortable but quite difficult to pinpoint the reason behind it.

My sister was a 'worried' mother before any problems were really encountered. Any incidents that have occurred since then have just heightened her worries but they have not been the cause of them. Before having children I looked forward to becoming a mother. I loved children and could not wait to actually have my own child – but I was not prepared for the overwhelming feelings of panic that arose when I realised that this little person's well being was completely down to me! To suddenly be aware that a person relied solely upon me was an immense amount of pressure – and I do not believe any woman is entirely ready for that. No matter how much babysitting practice they have 'under their belt' it is entirely different to be unable to hand that child back to someone else when you are tired and stressed.

Every new mother must be aware of the dangers of cot death. It is wise to strictly adhere to the guidelines that are in place at the time of your baby's birth – but to continue to check on your child's breathing, when they are well past toddler hood, must seem just a little over cautious. But I was so convinced that my child would die that I constantly had to check on him. It is easy to look for excuses. I had suffered a miscarriage with my first child - and threatened to miscarry my son - so my over zealousness can be explained by that. I often dismissed my feelings of impending doom as a bi product of the child I lost – but these feelings are not quite as simple as that.

I recall my sister advising me not to continually 'give in' to my son because I was not doing him any favours – but I had a dreadful feeling that he was going to die. The thought of losing him was bad enough but, the thought of losing him after I had told him off, or refused to give him something, was absolutely unbearable. I know I made plenty of mistakes with him, and continue to do so even today.

I feel that I must explain further about the dreadful feeling that he was going to die. This was not just a little niggling doubt that he would not survive baby and toddler hood – this was almost a 'premonition' that I was going to lose him. Losing a child is every parent's worst nightmare. I imagine every parent has experienced this worry – but I expect it is usually preceded by a valid reason. If your child is seriously ill, or hurt in a terrible accident, the possibility of losing that child is a very real one.

My sister tragically lost a child and her worry over her youngest son's well being could easily be put down to the trauma that was triggered by that loss. But, in truth, she had problems well before this incident.

ALL IN THE MIND

I am often accused of being 'too soft' when it comes to my children. I could use the excuse that the loss of my nephew had a profound effect on me - but that is all it would be: an excuse. It *did* affect me deeply but I was soft on my children well before that loss.

My fear of losing my children has lessened as they have grown up – but it has not diminished entirely. My pleas to 'be careful crossing the road' have now been shortened to simply 'be careful' – but if they are running late I still 'know' that they have been involved in a terrible accident and the police will be arriving at my door at any moment.

We tend to look for reasons and excuses to explain our behaviour. Although on the surface it looks like a valid explanation for the way in which we behave, if you look further back you will very probably discover that you were uncomfortable in certain situations, even before that 'major event'. What appeared to be the turning point in your ability to cope was simply the 'last straw'.

Beverly was never very happy waiting in queues at the post office. When she suffered a panic attack whilst waiting in line to be served, this became the reason for her disliking queues. But, the fact that she was uncomfortable even before that initial panic attack, seemed to evade her entirely.

Laura felt that she did not need to go out. She kept herself busy indoors and her husband was quite happy to do the shopping on his own. She enjoyed cooking and sewing and could always find plenty to keep her occupied – it was only when it was pointed out to her that she had not left the house in eighteen months, that she was made aware that she *did* have a problem. She denied feeling depressed but the fact that she had lost all interest in socialising was an important pointer. To people who go out on a regular basis this may seem quite bizarre that someone could feel 'happy' staying indoors day after day, night after night.

Human beings are social animals and it is generally a bad experience in a social setting of some kind that triggers feelings of inadequacy that sufferers are keen to avoid in the future.

Brea suffered problems at school, which resulted in her reluctance to stay on and take exams. It was more verbal bullying than actual violence that made her school life a nightmare. Years later, feeling stupid and inadequate, she enrolled at college where she was surprised to stand out as an excellent student. Years of feeling inferior made her unwilling to open up to her fellow students with the result that they began to view her as a bit 'above herself'. They were not above asking for her help – and she was not above giving it – but they made her feel less and less a part of the group until they ostracized her altogether. That, added to her previous experience at school, has done nothing to change her views on her fellow man. Is it surprising then that she avoids social contact now? Why would she want to put herself through that again?

ALL IN THE MIND

She was assured that there were some nice people out there – and that further education was the place for adults who actually wanted to improve themselves, and not school kids who were out to cause trouble. She plucked up the courage to enrol at college, only to be bullied in much the same way that she had been when she has still been at school.

It is a harsh fact of life that bullies in the schoolyard are more than likely to become bullies in the 'office' too. If someone has spent their formative years belittling and badgering other people then they are hardly going to stop that behaviour in later years, are they?

That said, many people *do* change. Some teenage rebels can come out the other side as nice human beings. The calming effect of having children themselves – and the realisation that they would hate anyone to hurt them – can have a remarkable effect on them. Of course this change of heart cannot be relied upon.

I suppose bullies have their own problems to contend with – maybe they are being bullied at home and this is the only way that they can regain some control of their lives? When they boss other people about and intimidate them, it makes them feel 'big and strong' as opposed to feeling 'small and weak' – the way they possibly feel at home? Whatever the reason, it does not excuse their behaviour – or excuse the fear and anxiety that they cause other people to feel.

ALL IN THE MIND

CHAPTER 13

We all worry from time to time. It is normal to worry about a new event that is about to happen – going for a job interview, starting a new job or going out on your first date with a prospective partner. But sometimes we worry out of context to the situation. If it is a normal event, and we are worrying ourselves sick over it, then this is not going to help us to cope in a new situation – but this realisation does not always help; in fact, it can simply make us feel worse.

Worry causes stress and this causes just as many physical problems as depression and phobias. When you worry it is all consuming – you are unable to take your mind off the problem and any effort to get you to 'stop worrying' may provoke a hostile reaction from you. A major cause of stress that has been in the news recently is work - related. We are all trying to fit so much into our lives that we are not able to cope with all the demands that we make upon ourselves.

One of the main symptoms of stress is insomnia. Sleeplessness on its own can cause a whole host of problems. The odd night or two can be hard enough to take – lack of sleep causes irritability and a lack of concentration to name but two – but prolonged bouts can be torture. And I am not exaggerating there – sleep deprivation was used as a form of torture in the war so its' effects should not be ignored. Insomnia can cause other physical problems – it lowers your immunity, making it far more difficult to fight off the usual coughs and colds – and the irritability and pressure it puts you under causes stress to build up, which increases the likelihood of your developing depression and phobias.

These symptoms can have a 'knock on' effect in the rest of your life. A lack of concentration can lead to mistakes being made and a 'bad mood' can set off a whole string of arguments that might have been avoided if you were well rested. Persistent coughs and colds go hand in hand with feeling generally run down and can make every day tasks look like enormous treks.

Trying to locate the cause of the problem is far more beneficial than simply resorting to taking sleeping pills - though I am not belittling their effectiveness on a short-term basis, or for prolonged insomnia, for which the usual remedies have been fruitless.

The usual remedies are, of course:

- ✓ Take a relaxing bath before bedtime – adding some essential oils, like Lavender, can be even more effective.
- ✓ Keep things like tea and coffee – or indeed anything containing caffeine – to a minimum – try and drink something milky instead.
- ✓ Avoid eating late at night – your digestive system will continue to work for a couple of

ALL IN THE MIND

hours after you have eaten so make an evening meal light.
- ✓ Exercise – I know how you feel, but this is supposed to release 'feel good' hormones that help you to relax. On the positive side, if you exercise you may exhaust yourself into falling asleep anyway, so there you have two reasons for having a go!

There are other physical ways that you can assist yourself. By creating the right atmosphere, you can also increase your chances of falling asleep. Sprinkling diluted essential oils onto your pillow or bedcovers – or using relaxing aromatherapy room sprays – can also aid you in your task. But, if there is more of a physical reason – a snoring partner or a street lamp right outside your bedroom window – then looking for ways to minimise these nuisances (like ear plugs and an eye mask) may improve your chances!

What if the problem is not falling asleep but *staying* asleep that weighs heavily on your mind? Do you fall asleep reasonably quickly only to wake up in the early hours and end up laying there thinking over the day's events – or simply worrying about tomorrow? It has been suggested that writing down your worries can prevent them from 'playing on your mind' and preventing you from sleeping – I have always believed in doing something constructive so I would recommend this as a first step, although I am not too sure how effective it would be.

If you are not the type of person who enjoys writing, then this in itself might create more problems than it solves. If you cannot write down your worries, try talking to someone. If you cannot think of anyone to whom you feel able to confide, look through the phone book for any suitable helpline to telephone. Talking to someone is a good idea, but for people who are unable to do this, maybe an alternative would be to speak into a cassette recorder. You could play it back and use yourself as a 'listener' to see if any solutions present themselves – or simply wipe it clean later. It is the act of talking the problem over, that is sometimes helpful in alleviating anxiety, and not the possibility of actually finding an answer to that problem. Experiment to see what works best for you.

If you feel unable to do that, then maybe you should consider visiting the doctor's surgery. Unless you can come to terms with your problems, that wonderful restful night's sleep is always going to elude you.

I mentioned writing above, and it is obvious that this is something that I enjoy. I have often been surprised when people hate to put pen to paper - but I know several people that loathe this to such an extent that they will even 'employ' other people to write out their Christmas cards! It is a hard admission to make that I write for enjoyment – having never had any of my work published, it is somewhat embarrassing too – and when I make

ALL IN THE MIND

this admission to an avid reader, I am even more surprised when they find it amazing.

I have always imagined that anyone who loves reading is bound to want to create their own masterpiece – and when I realise that they have no such desire, I simply cannot understand it. I have often explained that I love writing because anything can happen in my books. As a reader I may wish this or that would happen in a book, but as a writer, I am in charge of events.

In a programme recently, an author faced a diagnosis of illness which the physician explained he had to accept and that he had no control over it. Also, that although he was used to controlling everything in his books – right down to the weather – he was not in control of his health and he could appreciate how helpless that made him feel.

There is that control issue again.

CHAPTER 14

I mentioned the fact that I watch GMTV in the mornings in a previous chapter. Recently, they did a short series tackling phobias, and Hypnotherapist Paul McKenna made a guest appearance curing viewers of their ultimate fears. They advertised for people who had extreme fears or phobias to appear on the programme and picked several subjects throughout the week.

One lady was so afraid of enclosed spaces that she was unable to use a lift – by the end of her session she was able to spend a prolonged period of time nailed into a wooden crate: her claustrophobia miraculously cured. Another lady had spent years suffering with toothache - and had never taken her children to the see the dentist – because of her intense fear. By the end of her session she not only sat in the dentist's chair, she was calm enough to have the dentist examine her teeth! A gentleman who appears in a quartet featured on the Jonathan Ross show, was terrified of flying – only to be whisked around in a helicopter by the end of his session.

The climax of the week was an experiment to cure as many people of their phobias as possible – through the television screen. There were several sessions being held in various locations with the aid of Paul McKenna's assistants. There was a group of people being treated for their fear of heights, another group being treated for their fear of snakes

ALL IN THE MIND

and a group of arachnophobes being treated in Wales (the area, apparently, where there are more people battling with a fear of spiders than anywhere else!).

I am not that keen on heights, or enclosed spaces, but it was the last fear to which I could identify more readily. It was also the phobia to which I noted the most intense reaction. A group of women (and I have to admit that there seemed to be far more women suffering from extreme fears than men) literally ran away in tears when someone approached them with a tarantula crawling on the back of their hand. I found myself flinching away as well – and the television screen distanced me from it – but to see some of them, later, calmly allowing that same tarantula crawl to on *their* hand was amazing!

Paul McKenna insisted that anyone can be cured of their fears, it just takes longer to cure some people than others – and the results speak for themselves – but what if the fear that you have, is of people? By its very nature you are unable to seek help because it means approaching the very thing that you are afraid of! There were some hints and tips available though, and I feel that it is important to note them here.

Paul McKenna introduced a 'tapping' system that he had been shown by an American expert. He did not name this gentleman, so I am unable to do so here, but he states that it is a way to re-programme the brain. He informed us that we are born with only two fears – the fear of loud noises and the fear of falling – the rest we simply 'learn' to fear. If we can learn to fear something we can un-learn it. The brain, he says, is like a computer and can be re-programmed. This 'tapping' exercise is apparently an extremely effective way of doing that.

Think of the thing that you are afraid of and rate your fear from 1-10. 1 means that it only slightly bothers you, 10 means that it is unbearable. Whilst thinking of your fear, take two fingers (he used the pointer and middle finger of his right hand) and tap under one eye (top of cheek bone) a couple of times. (2 or 3 times seemed to be sufficient) but do it up to about 10 times to see how effective it can be.

Still thinking of your fear tap under one arm (bra strap level) and then just below your collarbone. Now tap the back of one hand and keep doing so whilst you carry out the following actions:

Close your eyes tightly and then open them.
Look down to the left then down to the right.

Then move your eyes as though you are looking around in a circle – first one way and then the other; (anti clockwise then clockwise or vice versa – I am not sure if it matters).
Count slowly, out loud, from 1-5.
 Now **hum** 'happy birthday to you, happy birthday to you, happy birthday dear whoever happy birthday to you'.

ALL IN THE MIND

Rate your fear again. Has it decreased at all? It apparently should have done so but, if not, go through the whole exercise again (right from tapping under one eye) and see if you can notice a difference.

If you are not very good at imagining your fear, see if you can find a picture or representation of it that you can cope with looking at. I know some people cannot even cope with seeing a photograph of a spider, so only use this method if you are able to do so. I suppose you could use the picture after attempting the 'tapping exercise' a few times to see how effective it has been in decreasing your fear.

Paul McKenna also recommends visualisation exercises. I believe that this entails imagining the thing that you are afraid of, in a 'comical' way – a spider wearing skates for example. I do not think that I am very good at this because I am never able to find seeing a spider, no matter how ludicrously 'dressed', as funny! He had also prepared a hypnotherapy session, on the GMTV website, that viewers could download to help them in a more intense way – but that was only available if you could access the Internet. It was very interesting on the whole, but I am not convinced that it would work for everyone.

This brings to mind another point. It is easy to imagine that good things only happen to other people – other people can cope, other people can be cured – that good things like that cannot happen to you. A positive attitude is all very well, but when your past experience has only gone to prove that bad things happen to you, it is difficult to change your point of view.

ALL IN THE MIND

CHAPTER 15

I have given plenty of examples of how people can seem to have the same problem yet, on further investigation, it becomes clear that they are affected differently. A strategy that helps one person to cope will make another person feel even worse.

I was reminded of this when talking to Ruth recently. Ruth has had 'bad nerves' for years and because of this has been unable to hold down a job. One of her major symptoms is that she cannot cope with a 'set routine'. This, of course, makes working difficult because she will feel ill when she has to do something on a regular basis – and work, by its very nature, requires a routine to be established.

Repetition raises her anxiety levels to such a degree that she needs to 'get away' from the situation. She can cope for a short while – but if something threatens to become a regular thing then she cannot cope with it. This may sound like she needs excitement and challenge on a daily basis, but that could not be further from the truth. To some degree she likes to know what is happening and when – she needs to be prepared – so it would not be accurate to describe her as spontaneous. Not being able to cope with a 'set routine' is not the same as enjoying the freedom to do as you please. A routine is just that: doing the same thing, at the same time, on the same day. If you have ever had a monotonous job you may be able to appreciate Ruth's inability to cope with the mundane.

Having a monotonous job may drive you to tears, it may bore you beyond belief, but does it make you incapable of doing it? It was not the job that Ruth could not do; it was the 'set routine' that she could not cope with. The getting up at a certain time, the physical act of getting to the job and the knowledge that she had to spend the next eight hours there – those were the issues that she could not face.

Ruth is not lazy. She keeps herself busy and she enjoys keeping fit. Her inability to get and keep a job has nothing to do with a lack of energy or a negative attitude. It has everything to do with her being unable to cope with a certain situation – with something that has been established as a routine.

Stacey, on the other hand, finds repetition comforting. To have a routine established – to know what she will be doing from day to day, week to week, - gives her a sense of security. It is only when changes occur that she feels unable to cope. Stacey can be bored doing various aspects of her job – but this does not change her view that, on the whole, she prefers to keep to her routine. To her mind, even knowing that she has to do a boring job, is a form of security. She is not keen on change.

Why does routine affect these people differently? Is it their attitude to boredom? One cannot cope with boredom whilst the other can? On the surface this seems a logical assumption – but it is not the

ALL IN THE MIND

boredom that Ruth cannot cope with is it? Ruth cannot cope with the routine.

To a certain degree I enjoy my routine. I look forward to the days that I do not have to go to work and can plan what I will do with my free hours whilst the children are in school. I guard my free time somewhat fiercely and can feel very low if I have to give it up.

I will generally avoid volunteering my free time, but have been asked to do various favours for other people, when they know I have a day off. Unless this impinges on my own plans, I am reluctant to refuse and end up spending my free time doing things I would generally prefer not to do. If this happened day after day, week after week I could very easily snap!

If I gave in to these requests on a regular basis, I can well imagine feeling very depressed, angry, resentful and anxious – not to mention put upon, taken for granted and downright fed up! I might very well think that I cannot cope with any more, and feel obliged to walk out.

This is the nearest I can get to imagining how Ruth feels. Maybe after years of raising her own family she now wants to protect her own free time as fiercely as I want to protect mine? Maybe if she is forced into a routine she feels that there is no escape from the monotony - and can think of better ways of spending her time? Ruth has raised her family and maybe that is the crucial point. She has 'finished' her job – and is still on hand to help out with the grandchildren. Why shouldn't she protect her free time as fiercely as I protect mine?

In an age where women have earned the right to equality, it seems quite ironic to state that I wish we could go back to the 'good old days' – but I do. It seems that the penalty for equal rights and equal pay is an increase in mental health problems. It seems that we are forcing each other to take advantage of all that is on offer in society today. Women are not just capable of working outside the home; today, they are expected to do so.

But women who take on paid jobs still have that other 'job' to do as well – that unpaid, unappreciated job that seems to fall on all women – that of 'Homemaker'. Whether or not a woman has young children to take care of, she is still the main person expected to clean, cook, wash dishes and do the laundry.

Is it any wonder that women suffer depression and stress at home as well as in the work place? But men do not have it easy in this area either. Man has long been established as the provider for his family – and, as such, has looked upon woman to care for his needs.

What we have today are women who are as capable of providing for their family as the men are - and they are looking to their mate to help care for their needs too – even if they are reluctant to voice them! A man is now expected to go to work and then come home and do his share too – which is only fair if his partner has also been working all day. But the majority of men still tend to view housework as a woman's domain and will only help out in certain areas.

I think that the lines have become blurred between male and female boundaries and I do not believe that this is altogether a good thing. I know that depression and stress have always existed but have they ever been as prevalent as they are now?

My mother was ill throughout my childhood, and I began writing this book with the fact that my father had a nervous breakdown when he was in his fifties. I also noted that my first indication of this was when he was washing the dishes and turned to face us in tears.

Did my mother's ill health, and the fact that my father had to take on 'her' role, play a key role in the deterioration of his mental health? Maybe this is just a coincidence but I feel it is a point worth mentioning just the same. I do not really think that I want the 'good old days' to resume. I was not around to see them the first time, so I am more than a little aware that they were probably anything but 'good'.

I also do not think that those who fought for equal rights for women would thank me for my views above either – but I am raising questions, rather than voicing an opinion, so I hope that they will not judge me too harshly. I guess that society needs to reassess its views as a whole. Choices need to be respected and this means that people should not be pigeonholed. If someone wants to work as well as raise a family then they should get all the support that they need. If they choose one or the other that choice should be respected too. Making choices is all about taking control – and I feel that that has been an important factor recognised throughout this book.

ALL IN THE MIND

CHAPTER 16

I have previously mentioned childhood and the impact it can have on how we behave as adults. Now I would like to discuss the possible impact our behaviour can have on our children. As a parent you have the overwhelming desire to protect your children. It becomes second nature to foresee hazards and put in place safeguards to ensure that your child does not get hurt. To avoid a dangerous fall we take the precaution of fitting safety gates to the top and bottom of the stairs, and safety plugs are inserted into electric sockets to prevent the possibility of electrocution.

These are typical safety measures and no one could accuse a parent of being over cautious for carrying them out. But what if you take safety measures too far? I have already admitted to being an overprotective mother and a worrier so it should come as no surprise that I am guilty of doing just that.

I bought my sons mobile phones just before they started secondary school. Prior to that they were not allowed far enough away from home to warrant using one – besides which they were provided with walkie talkies to ensure that they could reach me in an emergency! However, along with secondary school came the added necessity of going outside the walkie talkie range and so a mobile phone was purchased.

Some people might have viewed this as an unnecessary waste of money and an indication that I was giving in to peer pressure. However, it had more to do with my own feelings than it had to do with theirs. Feeling anxious when my children are out of sight can be an ordeal and the knowledge that I can contact them in an emergency, goes some way to relieving the stress. If I cannot get hold of them (if I do not have a signal or it goes straight through to voicemail) then I convince myself that they are hurt or injured and unable to call for help.

This may sound bizarre and silly but these feelings are very real. They are actually like premonitions. The vision is so clear that it is difficult to ignore. But how does this impact on my sons? Up to a point they understand how I feel and try to allay my fears. However, in recent years, my eldest son has felt a little resentful. His friends make fun of him when I call to check up on him, and this causes him some embarrassment. He sometimes fails to take his phone on purpose and then tells me that he forgot it!

My youngest son is very understanding. Too understanding really and that is down to the fact that he feels the same way himself. If he cannot get hold of me he starts to panic that I have been involved in an accident and am hurt. He gets very upset and I feel guilty that I have played a role in creating those feelings.

ALL IN THE MIND

It does not help that children and adults have been assaulted locally and gone missing nationally. Instead of thinking that we are safe we imagine that something awful has happened to each other. We are told to warn our children of 'stranger danger' but how far should we go? The trouble is children believe that they are immortal and can fight off any 'baddie'. I tell my sons that the first form of self defence is to run and I remind them that every person who has been kidnapped, or attacked, would have put up a fight so they should not rely on their strength to ward off an attacker.

Even with the realisation that you are far more likely to be attacked by someone you know than a stranger, it is hard to put that into perspective when you are unable to obtain an answer to your call. Trying to be sensible is just not possible. The fear in the pit of your stomach does not leave room for logic. You know something awful has happened and even when you are proved wrong it does nothing to lesson the fear next time.

It is sensible to put some safety measures in place and the fire service recommend that we all go through our own fire drills so that we know how we would get out of the house in an emergency. But what if you take this to the extreme and think of actions and reactions to the most bizarre events? We not only discussed fires breaking out in all parts of the house and the exits we would use in each case, but we would also go through throwing bedding out through the window, so we would have a soft place to land and when it would not be safe to try to locate each other. The boys were warned not to try to get to me, but to climb out of the window and lower themselves from the sill until they were hanging by their hands, before letting themselves drop to the ground.

They also liked to have a plan in place should anyone break in. Here I was not quite so worried and reassured them that the chances of that happening were slim as we lived in a terraced house. We would then discuss various houses lived in by our friends and relatives and devise plans should these more isolated buildings be broken into!

We would walk for miles when my children were younger and some of our walks took us on quite lonely routes. I would start feeling nervous and pick up a big stick or branch that could be used as a weapon and I would tell the boys what they should do if something happened to me. They would arm themselves with sticks too and it is quite sad that my nerves actually made mundane events seem quite adventurous!

It is little wonder that my youngest son is quite nervous still and is always prepared with a back up plan should something happen. He is always saying things like 'if we broke down here I'd do so and so', and 'If such and such happened I'd do this!'

Our children's health is another area where we can do untold damage. For most parents the threat

ALL IN THE MIND

of a serious illness will bring about all kinds of concerns and anxieties. For me, however, even the simplest thing could raise my anxiety levels. A headache could be meningitis, stomach ache could be appendicitis and a temperature could be the beginnings of something terrible! It is hardly surprising that I spent so much time in the local surgery that it would have been beneficial to book a room and a bed!

So, I can hardly blame my sons now when they fear the worst, can I? My eldest son fell off a go-cart and hit his side on a metal post. His skin was not even pierced, yet he was convinced that he had done irreparable damage to his liver! My youngest son suffers with abdominal problems and is certain that his appendices is about to burst! After years of worrying myself silly I am reassured that their ailments are not life threatening – but my worries and concerns have transferred themselves to my sons.

Richard believes that he is ill and convinces himself that he has any illness mentioned in his hearing. He will repeat 'parrot fashion' what he hears and convinces the doctor that these symptoms are real. Perhaps to him they are. To someone who has seen a lot of illness maybe he cannot believe that he has managed to escape 'scot-free' himself.

Gloria too convinces herself that she has had every illness in existence (and more besides) and has always experienced each illness worse than anyone else. She does have a real illness but rarely mentions that so why does she complain, so readily, about illnesses of which she is not a sufferer? Does she want pity? Does she want compassion? Does she really believe that she has suffered from all of these illnesses? Or is she 'making it all up'? If she truly believes that she has such poor health then maybe she should receive more sympathy that she does. However, her family have experienced years of her moaning about her ill health and now go into 'auto pilot' when she starts to complain about non existent illnesses.

It is not always easy to see beneath the surface and understand why someone behaves in the way that they do. Some people will moan about next to nothing whilst another will not mention some quite serious problem. Most of Gloria's children will avoid visiting the doctor at all costs – anxious not to be labelled as hypochondriacs – whilst the odd one will envisage that the slightest twinge is evidence of some sinister illness and needs constant reassurance.

People can refer to people like Gloria as hypochondriacs but this is actually an illness in itself. These people are not just making things up, they actually believe that they have the symptoms concerned and are therefore convinced that they suffer from the dreaded illness. It must be quite frightening to be bombarded by symptoms that you have read about and to be told that it is all in the mind. To the sufferer, the illness may not be real but the symptoms are very much so. And, like I

ALL IN THE MIND

pointed out in an earlier chapter, when something is 'all in the mind' it is in the very place where it can do the most damage!

CHAPTER 17

I mentioned in the previous chapter the fact that I am an overprotective mother who constantly worries about her children. You may imagine that I have always been that way so it may surprise you that I found it difficult to bond with my eldest son. A lot of mothers may find that a terrible admission to make and may assume that I did not want or love my son. But they would be wrong.

After losing my first child, my initial reaction on discovering that I was pregnant again, was one of dismay. I was convinced that I would miscarry my next child too and I did not feel that I could cope with that either physically or emotionally.

When I threatened to miscarry again I was 'proved' right. I felt scared, upset and anxious but, I also felt guilty. Why had I allowed myself to get pregnant again? Obviously I was unable to carry a baby and I felt that the initial miscarriage had been my fault (who else could have been to blame?). I also felt like a complete failure as a woman.

I was not reassured even when the scan showed a 'viable foetus'. I was still convinced that something awful was going to happen and was surprised when, after a few days of bed rest, I was allowed to return home. As my bump grew I felt more and more anxious. Instead of seeing it as a healthy sign of my baby growing and developing normally I saw it as a torment. I would lose the

ALL IN THE MIND

baby even later in the pregnancy and that would just make matters worse. I did not feel able to confide in other people because I knew that they would think I was 'going mad'. They may even think that I did not want my baby and it was 'wishful thinking'.

When labour started at 31½ weeks I was again 'proved' correct. The baby was 'small for dates' and it looked as though it was unlikely that he would survive the birth. I was terrified. Even though I had mentally prepared myself for this all along, I now felt that I could not cope. I begged them to stop the labour but they could not.

Labour stopped of its own accord and although I was relieved, I was waiting for the next thing to go wrong. I knew that I was going to lose this child, I just did not know when.

When he was born, within days of his original due date, he was a healthy 6lb 11oz. I should have felt ecstatic, relieved and overjoyed to have delivered a healthy baby. But I felt scared and overwhelmed. Instead of this being the end of the pregnancy it was the beginning of a baby's life that I was certain would end in a cot death.

Maybe it was because of the initial miscarriage that I still felt that I was not a 'normal' woman and therefore could not bring a healthy life into the world? I do not know. I just 'knew' that he was not going to survive and I was frightened that I was going to find his lifeless body in his cot one morning. 'Knowing' that this was going to happen made me reluctant to bond with him. I would feed him, change his nappy, wind him and nurse him but a part of me was determined not to get too attached.

It was as if I was telling myself that if I kept emotionally 'distanced' from him then it would not be as painful when he died. Of course, this did not work. The more I tried not to care, the guiltier I felt. If I left him to cry, how was that going to help? If he died I would be mortified that I had not 'loved him' enough. Losing him would be hard enough without the guilt of not having loved him enough.

This made the situation worse, as my initial conviction that he would not survive babyhood, did not fade away. As he got older, I would refrain from telling him off because I could not live with the guilt if he later died in his sleep. Of course he did not die but my fear that he would was very real and despite my feelings being wrong, I 'knew' he was going to die just as surely as I knew that day would follow night.

I have tried to explain why I felt the way that I did but maybe I am trying to find logic where there is none? I can only explain things from my perspective and try to make sense of it from that angle. As I have admitted previously, I am not a professional.

Violet found it difficult to bond for reasons that are perhaps easier to understand. She had given birth

ALL IN THE MIND

a month early and both she and her daughter almost died during the labour. There was no time for the baby to be placed upon her breast to bond before being whisked away to receive specialist care. Violet too needed specialist care and was too exhausted and groggy to consider how her daughter was doing. When she was finally allowed to see her she felt nothing. The tiny baby might just as well have been a plastic doll for all the maternal feelings that she was able to raise in her mother.

But why should this be either surprising or shocking? Labour is a very exhausting and difficult process for mother and baby and although most women are programmed to 'forget' the pain almost immediately, for others it is a very traumatic experience that they will never forget.

Hormones play an important part as they are 'all over the place' during the pregnancy itself; they then go through another change after the birth. Is it any wonder that some people are unable to connect with a tiny life that caused them so much pain only minutes earlier?

I remember reading about a man whose wife had died during childbirth. During his wife's last moments she had forced him to promise to take care of their daughter. He had assured her that he would but on seeing the baby all he felt was resentment and anger that she had been the reason that his wife had died.

As illogical as his thoughts may have been I believe that they are understandable. He loved his wife and they had both wanted this child. But the birth had been complicated and resulted in her death. If someone causes the death of a loved one it is natural to feel anger and resentment towards them.

The same is true of some men who are unable to bond with their child because they were present at the birth and remember the pain that was caused to their partner. Obviously a baby cannot be held accountable in these circumstances, but it gives an indication of how our human brains work. If a man can be 'forgiven' for being unable to bond immediately, then surely we can forgive ourselves if we take a little longer than what we believe is 'normal'?

Interestingly, the man kept his promise and grew to love his daughter more than he was able to express. He later considered her a 'blessing' and someone by whom he could remember his wife.

Some mothers are fortunate to fall instantly in love with their babies. For others the shock and trauma of the birth does not make this possible. It is the caring and nurturing of the baby that goes on afterwards, that creates the perfect opportunity for the bonding process to take place.

ALL IN THE MIND

CHAPTER 18

When I first started to write this account it was merely to close the gap between those who suffer with mental health problems and those who do not understand why someone can behave so irrationally. Along the way I have drawn my own conclusions and discussed my own theories on the possible reasons. But the more I consider the 'control' issue, the more convinced I am that this is more than just a coincidence.

Malcolm went through a 'bizarre' phrase where he spent ages putting away the shopping because all the canned goods had to be in neat rows with the labels facing to the front. It took him a considerable amount of time to organise it to his satisfaction and he would get quite agitated if the tins were disturbed. Now I am not talking 'Sleeping With The Enemy'- type agitated, but this is a control issue just the same. A little while later his wife found it satisfying herself and had to agree that it did look 'nice' and it made it easier to see what was in stock and what needed to be added to the shopping list.

To a certain degree I can accept this – it does look neater and there is something therapeutic in lining all the baked beans tins into nice, straight rows – but we are back to the realisation that we tend to rationalise our behaviour to make it more acceptable. I do not think that placing the canned goods into neat rows is, in itself, a problem. But the feelings it can produce, if the sufferer is not permitted to carry out the task, *are* a problem.

Friends and family members can then be drawn into the situation because they try to avoid the distress caused to their loved one. It is easy to dismiss 'minor' incidents but when does something become a major problem? If it affects your life, to the point where you avoid situations that might possibly have an adverse affect, then it is a problem. If you *have* to place those tins one behind the other, in order to feel 'safe', then maybe you need to look at the cause.

No one but you can know how you feel. A counsellor may be able to make you think about issues that you had not considered - but they cannot answer the big questions that *you* can. Why does your life feel like it is spiralling out of control? Why do you feel it is necessary to complete tasks, and in a certain order, to validate yourself?

You may be reading this expecting to find answers. Well, I am sorry to disappoint you. What you will probably do is ask yourself even more questions. This is not a self-help book or a promise that you will get better after reading it. I am simply trying to understand my own situation and if it helps others understand theirs in the process, then all the better.

I want people to realise that anyone can develop a mental health problem and just because they are fortunate enough not to suffer at present, they should not assume that they will never be affected. I wanted to put my fears and anxieties into words and phrases that anyone can understand. I wanted to explain what it is like to suffer irrational fears and try to give an insight into how frustrating it is to know that they are irrational - and yet to still be afraid. I do not want to encourage pity – self or otherwise. I want to encourage hope. If it helps you to realise that there are other people, out there, who understand how you feel then that is a positive result. If this helps one person to understand how their friend or loved one feels then that is an even better result.

It can be a very isolating illness. Our brains are unique to us and no one else has the power to read our thoughts or understand exactly how we feel. It is easy to describe a pain or diagnose chicken pox – but your mind is more personal. Even if several symptoms described here seem to be 'you' – they may affect you differently. The reason I feel the way that I do is personal to me – your reasons will be personal to you. But I think that if you can begin to understand the possible causes in your own life, it will help you to deal with them.

That is not to say that it will make all your problems go away. I feel that I understand myself better now but that does not stop me from hanging out the washing any differently. I just feel that understanding why you do something is another way of having an element of power over your life.

Being at the mercy of your problems is like being a martyr to them. It does not make you a weak person to realise that you have an issue. If you have a problem and have found the courage to admit it, then that makes you a stronger person. It may not make the problem any less of an issue but it does diminish its hold on you.

I am afraid of spiders. Telling myself I do not have a problem with them is only kidding myself – the moment I see one I will run from it (probably in tears depending on its size!) so to pretend that I can deal with them is futile. Admitting that I am afraid of them does not make me weak. It empowers me to joke about my fear and bring it down to size.

I have mental health problems. Admitting that, does not make me less of a person. It does not make me weak. I can joke about it and pretend that it has no power over me – that is easy to do when you are going through a good spell. You can distance yourself from it and see it for the irrational behaviour that it is. Tomorrow I may not be able to laugh about it but that makes me even more determined not to lose my good days to 'what ifs'. Laughter, as I say, is essential. I am having a good day, today, and I can cope.

I eventually managed to go to the doctor's surgery and ask for help with my anxiety problems. They cannot actually treat it when it occurs – I was advised to take medication now and see if it helps. The medication is used to treat depression as well

ALL IN THE MIND

so hopefully it will kill two birds with one stone. I was reluctant to take it so was given a very low dosage.

I am actually feeling pretty good at present. I am not sure if the medication has kicked in or if I was due to feel better now anyway – but I am feeling more positive and that is a good start. I have answered the telephone several times lately and did not feel too anxious. There was still an underlying feeling that, given a choice, I would prefer to let it ring - but I answered it anyway. The knowledge that I will be able to cope sometimes better than others, is bittersweet.

I accept that there are always going to be times when I will see the glass as 'half empty'. Those are the times when I will find it difficult to see the light at the end of the tunnel and the future will look bleak. And there will be times when I ask myself 'If I am this bad now, how bad will I be in the future?' But, I prefer to look at things in a more positive light - I am more of a glass 'half full' type of girl rather than a glass 'half empty' one – so I like to dwell on the times I can do things rather than the times I cannot.

We all have good days and bad days – and we all have our 'little quirks'. It is only the degree to how much those 'little quirks' affect our lives that give us the label of having a mental health problem. "If you can keep your head when all around are losing theirs ... then you evidently do not understand the problem!"

CONCLUSION

My main objective has been to give understanding to an illness that defies logic. I hope that the situations portrayed have given an insight into the possible feelings that a loved one has felt or, if you are a fellow sufferer, that you feel a little less isolated. Although it may be impossible to read another person's mind, or understand entirely how they feel, I hope that it has at least given you food for thought and has worked to make you a little less judgmental when confronted with mental health issues in the future.

It has been therapeutic to put my feelings into words and to try to attribute those same feelings to other people's situations. There is a proverb about 'walking a mile in another man's shoes' and I hope that I have given you the opportunity of at least trying on those shoes for a little while.

Mental illnesses are embarrassing and this causes the sufferer to feel isolated. To realize that you are not suffering alone can be a huge comfort. We are all human beings programmed with the same capacity to feel emotions like everyone else does. Even if we cannot understand why someone feels the way that they do, we should at least endeavour to validate their feelings and accept that although the problem may not be a 'real' one, the feelings that the problem creates are.

ALL IN THE MIND

It may be all in the mind but, as I have stated previously, that is the very place where it can do the most damage.

www.ingramcontent.com/pod-product-compliance
Ingram Content Group UK Ltd.
Pitfield, Milton Keynes, MK11 3LW, UK
UKHW041412180426
11947UKWH00007B/79